The Soldier's Foot and the Military Shoe

A HANDBOOK FOR OFFICERS AND NON-COMMISSIONED OFFICERS OF THE LINE

BY

EDWARD LYMAN MUNSON, A. M., M. D.
Major, Medical Corps, United States Army.

President, Army Shoe Board; Director, Field Service School for Medical Officers, The Army Service Schools, Fort Leavenworth, Kansas.

---

54 ILLUSTRATIONS

Approved by the War Department.

PREFACE

In the investigation of the Army Shoe Board, which extended over four years and included the critical study of the feet of some two thousand soldiers, the fitting of many thousands of pairs of shoes, and many months of direct inquiry into the causes affecting the shoeing of the United States soldier, it became evident that in very many instances the faulty conditions found were due to lack of information on this important subject on the part of the officers and noncommissioned officers of the line concerned.

The purpose of this book is to supply the practical information on this subject which has not heretofore been available, and without which it cannot be expected that the several factors which must correlate in order to produce the best foot conditions and marching capacity among American troops will be suitably recognized and satisfactorily coordinated.

To Captain William J. Glasgow, General Staff, and First Lieutenant Benjamin F. Miller, 27th Infantry, who, with the author, composed the Shoe Board, and to Captain John R. R. Hannay, 22d Infantry, later added as an additional member, very many of the new points here brought out on the subject of the military foot and footwear must be attributed.

THE ARMY SERVICE SCHOOLS,
FORT LEAVENWORTH, KANSAS,
JULY 31, 1912.

E. L. M.

CONTENTS

CHAPTER I.

FOOT INJURIES AND MARCHING CAPACITY.

It will not be disputed that the marching powers of foot troops are a most important factor in the conduction and success of battles and campaigns, and that the army which marches best, other things being equal, is the successful army. Mobility is the key of military success, and troops which cannot march will not be given, by a more vigorous enemy, opportunity to fight except under what may prove to be decisive military disadvantage. History is full of instances where military success has been won more by marching than by fighting, and as time goes on rapidity of movement will probably be an even greater element in military strategy in wars of the future than it has been in the past. The advantage of position, by which both the disadvantage of inferior force may be minimized and the power of superior strength still further enhanced, is the object of every commander.

Furse, in his "Art of Marching" says: "Marching is the foundation of all operation in war. An army below the standard in marching power is at the mercy of a more mobile force. Actual battle consumes but a fraction of the time spent in marching. The most brilliant plans fail if the troops do not march the distances calculated upon. Mobility is the first requisite of the soldier".

Napoleon is reported to have said that he made war not so much with the arms as the legs of his soldiers, while Forrest defined the art of war as "getting there first with the most men". Many examples could be given where battles have been lost and won by marching capacity. Waterloo was lost and history changed because of delay in the arrival of the expected French reinforcements—while the march of Jackson's socalled "foot cavalry" in the Manassas campaign of 1863 turned Pope's anticipated victory into the defeat of the

Second Bull Run. War has become a business in which each unit has its part to play; and the soldier whose badly shod feet are unable to carry him into battle fails at the critical moment of the purpose for which he was trained, and instead of being an added strength he becomes an incumbrance.

The effect of badly fitting shoes upon the psychology of war is very great. Even where the soldier is able to continue the march, the discomfort produced at every step soon reduces buoyancy of spirit, causes mental irritability and materially diminishes fighting capacity. As the attention and interest of the soldier is focussed upon his own personal condition and withdrawn from matters relating to the success of the military enterprise as a whole, the mental force which inspires the command to military achievement is dissipated and lost.

Some foot defects are in the nature of deformity in the anatomical relations of the foot structures. These mechanically weaken the foot and prevent it from exerting its powers to best advantage in the propulsion of the body in marching. Pain, also, may accompany these foot deformities and seriously interfere with marching power. Blisters and other injuries of the feet, which in themselves may be of no importance, require rest for their recovery. For this reason, they possess a very great practical interest from the military point of view, since they rapidly render a large number of men unfit for service and so diminish in large proportion the effective force relied upon at the beginning of a campaign.

The amount of disability from foot injury in modern armies is enormous. Brandt calculated that seven per cent of conscripts annually drafted for the German army are found unfit for military service by reason of foot defects due to bad shoeing. Lindau found that of ten thousand men discharged annually from the German army for physical disability in time of peace, four hundred were for affections of the feet—a proportion which he states would be tremendously increased in time of hostilities. In the early part of the Franco-Prussian War, in the Tenth Army Corps, the constant ineffectiveness from injury to the feet as a result of marching ranged from eight to ten per cent; and it is said that at one time not less than thirty thousand German soldiers were, from this cause alone, incapacitated for field service.

Léques found that excoriations of the feet figured as one-third of all the causes of exemption from active service among young French soldiers in campaign. In our Civil War, whole brigades were said to have been temporarily disabled and prevented from marching from this cause. Germaine has estimated that, after several days marching, about one-fourth of an infantry command would present excoriations of the feet and not less than ten per cent of the command would be in the hands of the surgeon; while military statistics in general show that from one-fourth to one-third of a command sustains foot injury in the first few days' marching. It has been estimated that for European armies an average loss of ten per cent must be expected from this cause among unseasoned troops on taking the field.

Examples of such incapacity and losses in our own army in more recent times are not wanting. Probably not an individual of any extended military experience but can recall instances in which the capacity of his command for marching was greatly diminished, and its effectiveness as a fighting force materially impaired, as a result of foot injuries. Many examples might here be cited, but the following instance which occurred in the experience of the Shoe Board is sufficiently typical.

In 1908, a battalion of United States infantry took a practice march in shoes which the men had themselves selected. It marched eight miles, went into camp for twenty-four hours, and then returned by the same route to the post. The members of the board examined the feet of all the men of the battalion at the end of the first day and again on their return. On the first day, 30 per cent, and on the last day 38 per cent, of the command were found to have severe foot injuries, some requiring hospital treatment. The feet of many others were reddened and sore from this short march, and a few more miles of marching would have converted these painful areas into blisters, and small blisters into large ones. This march is illuminative of what may be expected in our service if the matter of shoes and shoe fitting is turned over to the men and the matter of shoe supply is not given the attention its importance deserves.

But because foot injuries have usually been so common among soldiers of all armies is no reason for our accepting them with patient resignation as one of the inevitable concomitants of field service. The opposite is in fact the case. It is of grave military concern that the mere act of mobilizing a large military force by marching may require the immediate temporary discount of some ten per cent, of those previously effective, from foot injury. A cause which operates—without any possible compensating results—in practically every command at the beginning of a campaign to bring about the absence on the firing line of as many men as would be lost to that command as the result of a pitched battle is worthy of far more careful and thorough investigation than it has heretofore received. Inquiry shows that the armies of different countries are not alike—and within the same army its various component organizations may be quite dissimilar—in this respect. Moreover, it has happened that troops have been put into proper shoes and marched under field service conditions over long distances without the slightest loss from a cause which usually operates so severely. These exceptions, few and isolated though they may be, are proof positive that the general rule is the result of conditions which are unnecessary or removable. It thus becomes evident that proper care relative to the feet and shoes of infantry soldiers will be well recompensed by the increased efficiency of the latter. Since it appears that disability from foot injury can be prevented, it becomes a military duty to apply at all times the measures which it can be demonstrated will accomplish prevention.

In this connection, a brief summary regarding a recent march by regular infantry will be instructive. In this test march, which was conducted by the Shoe Board to try out the several military shoes, three types of the latter were employed, viz: the garrison tan shoe, the marching shoe of 1912 contracts, and the military shoe devised by the board. Enlisted men were fitted with a pair of one of these types—in regular sequence and irrespective of their preferences or desires, as the purpose was to determine and compare the respective effects of these different shoes upon the foot of the soldier class as a whole. But within each class, fittings were made as accurate and comfortable as possible. A full supply of all sizes and widths of each of these varieties of shoes was available for fitting. Eight companies participated in the march, and in each company about one-third the men had the same kind of shoe. The latter were worn by the men from twelve days to two weeks before the march, so as to get the feet reasonably habituated to the shape of the shoe supplied. Light wool socks were used for fitting and marching. The march included nine marching days; while the distance covered scaled 117½ miles but was probably at least 120 miles from bends and inequalities of the terrain. The shortest march was 8 miles; the longest 21 miles. A total of 379 officers and men, of whom 44 per cent were recruits of less than six months service, started on the march and 352 completed it. The full equipment, with ammunition, was carried. Not a single man failed to complete each day's march as a result of foot injury; losses from the command being due to a few cases of illness and accident and detachment for other duty on orders from higher authority. The feet of each man were inspected by the board after each day's march, and even the slightest pinhead blister was noted on the man's record card. Many of the injuries so reported were so trivial that at inspection on the following day they were not apparent and even their former location could scarcely be determined. This demonstration of the fact that it is quite possible to march American troops long distances without appreciable loss from foot injury is in marked contrast with the heavy loss which has habitually occurred under similar conditions in our own and other armies. The result justified the belief long held by, the board that any of the shoes as furnished by the Quartermaster's Department were fairly satisfactory, and that shoe difficulties and foot injuries heretofore obtaining in our army were chiefly due to shortage in the supply of sizes and widths of shoes available to troops through post quartermasters, and to ignorance, indifference and neglect on the part of company commanders in respect to the fitting to the feet of their men with such shoes as were available. Only such personal attention was given by the board to fitting as might reasonably be required of organization commanders and only such simple measures of foot cleanliness and care were carried out as could be enforced by the latter. Such trifling injuries as occurred, chiefly developed during the first few days when the men's feet were tender; and after the long 21 mile march, which was quite a severe test of the feet and endurance of the command. The percentage of recruits who developed foot injury was slightly less than that of the old soldiers, showing that length of service is not necessarily the important factor that it has heretofore been generally regarded, and that the higher proportion of recruits who in the past have probably had foot injuries was probably due to the difficulty in fitting themselves, with shoes of a new shape, in the sizes and widths to which they had been previously accustomed. In the entire march, 190 men, or 56.5%, never at any time suffered the most trifling injury of the feet; while 43.5% at one time or another suffered an appreciable lesion ranging from a pinhead blister undiscernable the next day to those of slightly larger size. Practically not a single injury of those which occurred was either large or severe. It thus appears that a very large proportion of the foot injuries common to marching troops, in number, extent and gravity, are unnecessary, are preventable by simple measures, and should be so prevented.

CHAPTER II.

THE ANATOMY AND USE OF THE FOOT.

The human foot is not to be regarded, as seems almost to be the idea with many, as an incoordinating mass of flesh, bone and gristle which may with impunity be crowded into almost any sort of protective covering to form a fleshy peg, more or less similar to a horse's hoof, on which to walk. It is, on the contrary, one of the most intricate anatomical structures of the human body. Every one of its parts has a definite function, and interference with its normal anatomical relations and development produces a corresponding structural defect or weakness which will always to some extent diminish—and not rarely is completely destructive of—the capacity to accomplish military marching.

Officers of the mounted branches are carefully instructed in the anatomy of the horse, with special attention to the hoof, foot and their related structures. For the cavalryman, it is appreciated that a competent knowledge of the inter-relations and coordinate functions of bone, muscle and sinew form an essential to the proper care and shoeing of the feet of his mount. This truth applies with even greater force to the soldier's foot; which in its structural anatomy is far more complex and delicate than that of a horse or mule, and in addition is compelled to wear a protection which, if poorly fitted, is much more liable to produce marching disability in the man than it is in the animal. It is impossible to effectively select and adapt a proper military shoe without a sufficiently comprehensive and intelligent knowledge of the integral and coordinating structures of the soldier's foot which is proposed to cover; yet study of the elementary regional anatomy of the human foot by all officers—including those specially concerned with dismounted troops—seems to have been practically disregarded in our service. It is of course not necessary that

Fig. 2

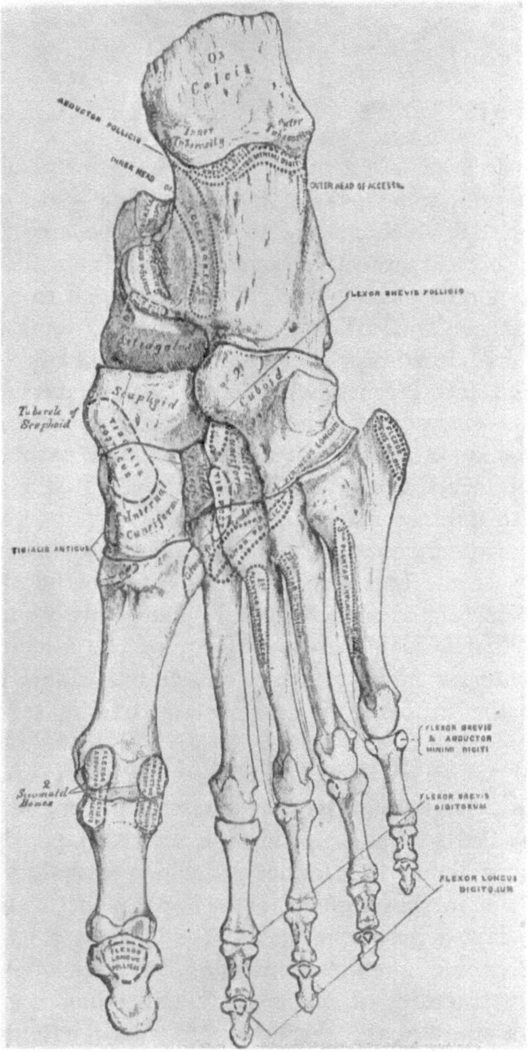

Skeleton of right foot, seen from below. (From Gray's Anatomy.)

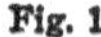

Fig. 1

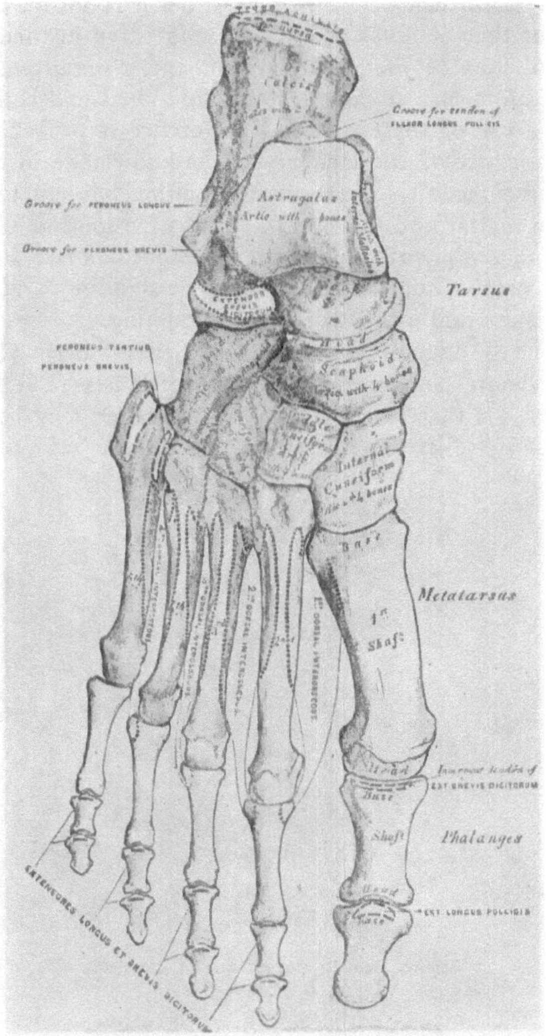

Skeleton of right foot, seen from above. (From Gray's Anatomy.)

line officers should go into minor details in this respect, or learn confusing medical terms; but it is not too much to expect that they should at least gain and carry in their minds a general idea of the nature of the more important structures of the foot and ankle, with the individual and collective purpose and use of these parts. Indifference is probably not so much the cause of the lack of proper knowledge in this respect, as is the fact that appropriate attention has not been directed to the matter and the necessary information has not been readily available in suitable form. The foot has two functions: That of passive support of the body in standing, and use as a lever to raise and propel the body in walking.

The human foot has as its general basis a framework or skeleton, composed of twenty-six bones (See Figures 1 and 2). Of these, nineteen are the so-called long bones, composed chiefly of hard, firm bony tissues, of smooth surfaces and

Fig. 3

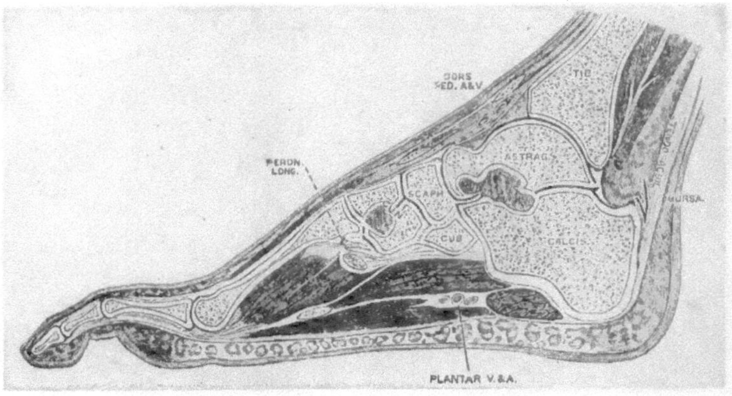

Section through foot on line of great toe. (From Volsz.)

various sizes, and joining with other bones at their ends only. The remaining seven bones, of various sizes, are composed of bone which is loose and spongy in texture; these bones have the appearance of irregular pebbles, and have many smooth facets forming surfaces for joining with adjacent bones, by which each bone is in contact with from four to six others. Fourteen of the long bones above mentioned are small and belong to the toes, while the other five are much longer and form the metatarsus or ball of the foot. The seven irregular and spongy bones form the basis of the foot arch and heel (See Figs. 3 and 4). One of these—the astragalus—articulates with the leg bones to form the ankle joint (See Figs. 3 and 4).

The heel is obviously intended by nature, through both position and structure, to receive the shock of impact of the foot against the ground and support the greater part of the weight of the body and burden in standing and at the beginning of a new step. (See especially Figs. 3 and 4). The os calcis, or heel bone, lies almost in prolongation of the line of the center of gravity of the body as represented by the leg bones. It is the largest bone of the foot, is broad and strong, and articulates closely with the astragalus—which lies above and in front of it and forms the keystone of the foot arch. The rear prominence of this heel bone is the point of attachment of the tendon of powerful muscles of the calf of the leg, which by their action lift the heel and rear of the foot off the ground and thus accomplish the first movement of the foot in walking. (See Fig. 3). This heel bone is guarded against injury by an especially thick layer of skin, fatty and fibrous tissue and muscle (well shown in Figs. 3 and 4), which serve as an efficient cushion between it and the ground. It is held firmly in position and attached to the bone it articulates with (the astragalus), and with other bones anterior

Fig. 4

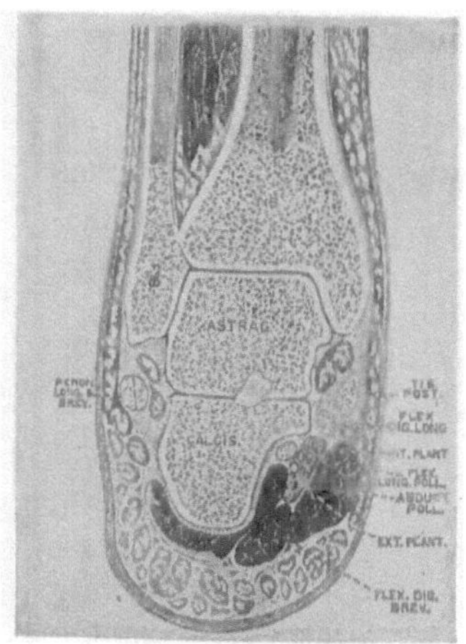

Transverse vertical section through ankle joint. (From Volsz.)

to it, by numerous strong ligaments and fibrous tissue (See Figs. 6 and 7). These attachments and the nature of the articulations of this bone permit of a certain degree of elasticity without true joint motion. The foot articulates with the bones of the lower leg, forming the ankle joint, through the astragalus. The latter also forms the keystone of the foot arch (See especially Figs. 2 and 7), as it is wedged between the heel bone and the scaphoid bone. It is a large, strong bone, with broad articulating surfaces, in contact with those of the leg bones, which embrace it on each side and support the entire weight with every step. From its position in the foot, its direct ligamentous attachments to other bones are relatively weak, but it receives additional support from the strong ligaments attached to other bones at the ends of the foot arch by which the latter are held together and prevented from spreading—and the astragalus from being thereby forced down—under the body weight. (See Figs. 6 and 7).

The front of the foot arch is formed by the five small bones, viz: the scaphoid, the cuboid, and the three cuneiform bones, together with the five metatarsals. The first five small foot bones are so closely articulated with each other by irregular surfaces, and are so firmly bound together by numerous small ligaments, as to form a compact bony mass, which is, however, capable of a certain limited amount of yielding under pressure which materially assists in lessening the shock to the foot and body which accompanies each step in marching. (See Figs. 6 and

Fig. 5

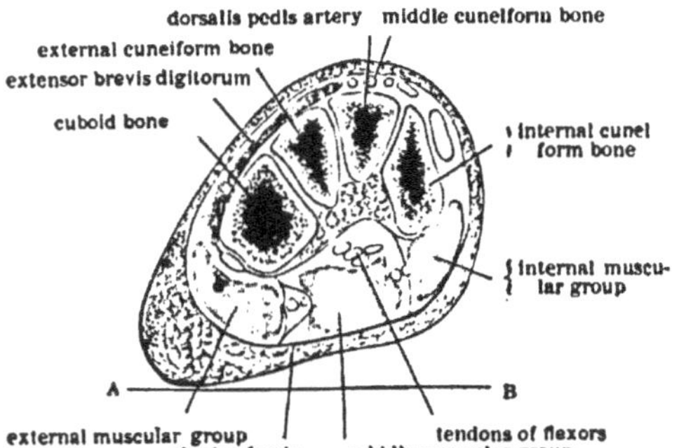

The Transverse Arch of the Foot. Section through the anterior row of tarsal bones. The line *A B* represents the surface upon which the foot rests when the individual stands erect. (From Gray's Anatomy.)

7). It will also be seen (Fig. 5) that the bones of this region not only form part of an arch extending from front to rear but also are so disposed among themselves as to form a secondary foot arch from side to side, thereby materially adding to the strength of the whole. Support to this lateral arch is given by ligaments and the tendon of one of the leg muscles.

From the very slight amount of elasticity and extremely limited relaxation anatomically possible as a result of the relations of the seven round bones of the foot, it is evident that a foot covering can logically be a close fit back of the tarso—metatarsal joint without in any way interfering with the purpose and functions of the foot.

The five long metatarsal bones form the extreme front of the foot arch. (See Figs. 1, 2 and 3, and all radiographs). They are firmly held at their posterior ends by ligaments binding them to the round bones of the foot (See Figs. 6 and 7), but the joints so produced are more flexible than those further back in the foot and permit of considerable motion downward (See Fig. 3). But between the shafts of these metatarsals there is no ligamentous union whatever, thus permitting marked spreading of these bones with broadening of the foot under pressure in the interests of greater flexibility, the production of broader surfaces and resulting increased stability in standing and marching. (See Fig. 6 and all radiographs). The frontal ends of these metatarsal bones, especially the ends of the first and fifth metatarsals, form the front of the foot arch (See Figs. 2 and 3). It will be noted (See Fig. 2) that the line of junction of the five metatarsals with the round bones of the foot, which forms the ball, is not square across but extends obliquely from without inward. The result of this oblique articulation, when the foot is pointed to the front, is to naturally tend to throw the weight of the body on the outer part of the foot, where the structures are strongest. The ball measurement in fitting shoes is taken just in front of this line of articulations, over the bony prominences at the base of the little and of the greater metatarsal bones.

This marked physiological capacity for spreading of the

metatarsal bones, especially at their anterior ends, together with that obviously possible in the unconnected toes, results in a requirement that any shoe suitable for military purposes shall be of such form and width in its anterior part as to allow proper broadening of the foot in its metatarsal and toe regions to the extent naturally assumed by the bare foot in standing and walking. If this be not done, the foot is narrowed, contact with the ground is decreased, and body equilibrium is impaired. In the natural effort to preserve the latter in too narrow shoes, the man tends to turn his toes out, thereby largely shifting weight from the strong outer margin of the foot so as to fall over the relatively weak inner arch.

Fig. 6

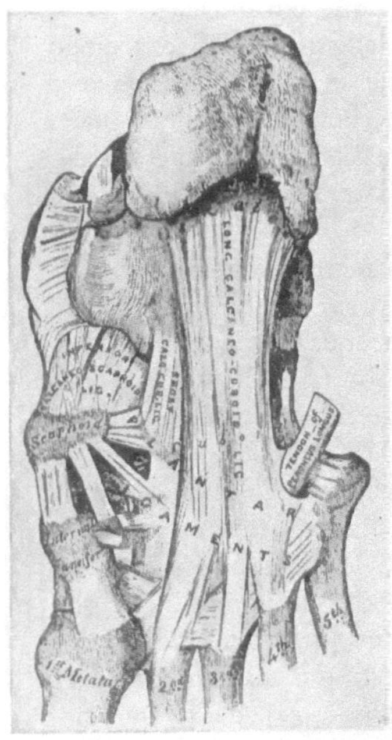

Ligaments of sole of foot. (From Gray's Anatomy.)

The bones of the phalanges or toes (See Figs. 1 and 2) articulate with their respective metatarsals, and with each other, in the production of joints intended to have a large degree of upward and downward mobility. This mobility of the toes is naturally greater than that of the fingers of the hand, with all the delicacy of use required of the latter, yet it is completely lost sight of by the average shoe manufacturer. Under pressure and confinement from ill fitting shoes, these highly mobile joints may largely or completely lose their function and the toes their use. Nearly all the muscles of the foot have their anterior attachments to the phalangeal bones or metatarsals, and contraction of these muscles causes the toe to press against the ground while lifting the body, near the end of the step, by pulling the ends of the foot arch nearer together and thereby increasing its concavity downward.

The resting position of the weight bearing foot is maintained by the ligaments, which are not elastic and are not overstretched in the normal foot. These ligaments bind the bones of the foot together. They hold up the foot arch only in the sense that they interfere at a certain point to prevent further spreading and flattening of the foot arch as a result of downward pressure.

Fig. 7

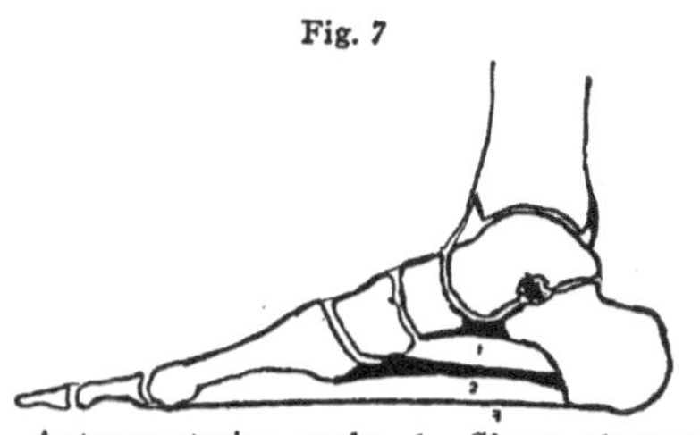

Anteroposterior arch: 1, Short plantar ligament; 2, long plantar ligament; 3, plantar fascia.

The manner in which the bones of the foot are bound together by these ligaments, which are the strongest of those in the body, is well shown in Figs. 6 and 7. These ligaments are tough, fibrous and inelastic, and are not intended to give much play to the parts they hold together. It will be observed that while these ligaments are numerous and run in all directions, by far the strongest ones—and those which naturally have to stand the greatest strain—are those which extend from front to rear of the foot arch. It will also be observed that while the sole of the foot is strongly bound together by ligaments, the latter are practically absent (See Figs. 3 and 6) on the upper part of the foot. The practical result of this location and arrangement of ligaments is that the natural tendency of the arch to flatten under pressure is checked at a certain point; while the absence of ligaments from the upper part of the foot permits of its flexion downward, with raising of the foot arch and a shortening of the distance between the heel bone and the metatarsals as the result of muscular contraction in walking. The relaxation or giving way of these ligaments is necessary in order that flat foot may occur.

But the passive resistance to pressure offered by the ligaments of the sole of the foot is not of itself sufficient to prevent flattening of the arch. Inelastic structures will ultimately tend to yield to excessive pressure which is sufficiently long continued. To provide against this, nature has reinforced these ligaments with an array of foot muscles, whose elastic contractions in producing locomotion also serve to take up a large part of the tension due to body weight which would otherwise fall directly on the ligaments. The intricate relations of these muscles to bones, ligaments and each other is clearly brought out in Figs. 8, 9, 10, 11 and 12. It will be observed from Fig. 3 that the muscles of the upper part of the foot, which are chiefly concerned in the slight labor of lifting the toes and fore foot, are few in number and of very slight development. However, one muscle of the leg—the tibialis anticus—has its attachment (See Fig. 2) on the under part of the foot arch, and by its contraction operates to heighten and hold up the latter. The muscles of the sole of the foot, on the contrary, are numerous and should be well developed and strong. Not only do they exert necessary tension, but they cushion the more delicate part of the foot and serve to protect it against injury. It will be observed from Figs. 8 to 12 inclusive, that there are no less than five distinct layers of muscles of the foot, practically all of which—except the transversalis muscles (See Fig. 10)—extend from the rear of the foot to its front. The outer or first layer of sole muscles (See Fig. 8) practically runs from the heel to the tips of the toes, their contraction resulting in flex-

Fig. 8

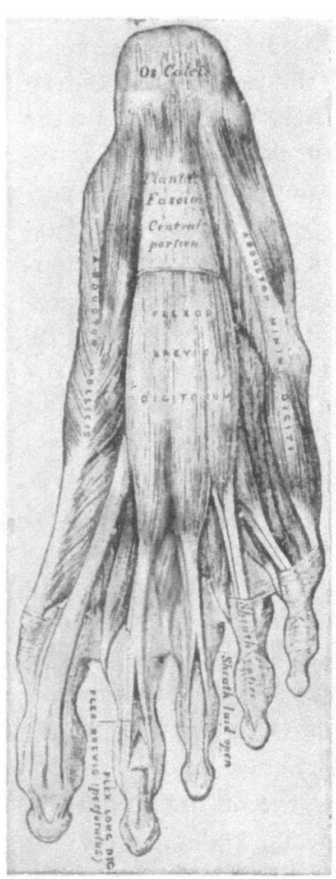

Muscles of the Sole of the Foot, first layer. (From Gray's Anatomy.)

ion of the foot and toes between these two points. The second layer of muscles (See Fig. 9) runs from the heel to the base of the toes, reinforced by the tendons of certain muscles of the calf of the leg. The third layer of muscles (See Fig. 10) strengthens the metatarsal region and adds additional force to the thrust of the ball of the foot against the ground in walking. The fourth and fifth layers of muscles, (See Figs. 11 and 12) with one group of the third, simply serve to prevent too great expansion outward of the smaller metatarsal bones in marching and assist in maintaining the balance of the body. The contraction of all these muscles flexes the sole, adducts the foot and forces the arch to rise. A buffer is thus formed which breaks the shock of impact of the ball of the foot against the ground.

Fig. 9

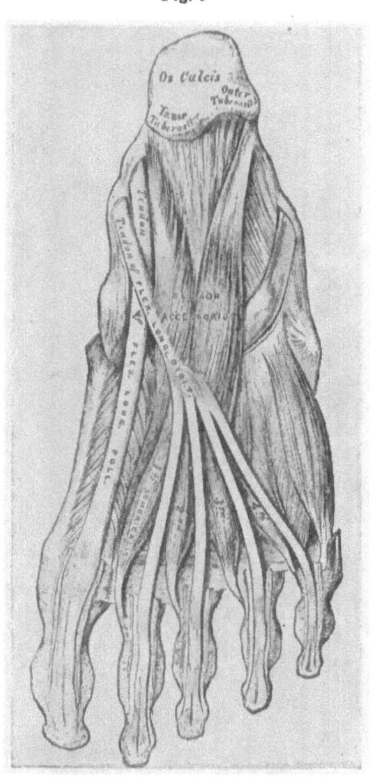

Muscles of the Sole of the Foot, second layer. (From Gray's Anatomy.)

The tendons of muscles operating on the sole of the foot are well protected and are not liable to incur injury. Those on the top of the foot, and particularly the one lifting the great toe, are superficial, are thinly covered with soft tissue, and lie directly over bones against which they may be pressed by too tight shoes, with resulting injury and inflammation of the tendons and fibrous sheaths in which they work.

Arteries, veins and nerves are of less practical importance in a study of the anatomy of the foot in relation to the shoe.

The arterial system lies fairly deeply between muscles and tendons, and pressure sufficient to materially affect it would cause such immediate discomfort as to bring about prompt remedy. The same applies to the nervous system. The veins, however, lie more superficially and may be pressed upon, particularly by shoes too tight around the ankle, sufficiently to cause more or less interference of the return flow of the blood with swelling of the foot below the point of compression.

Fig. 10

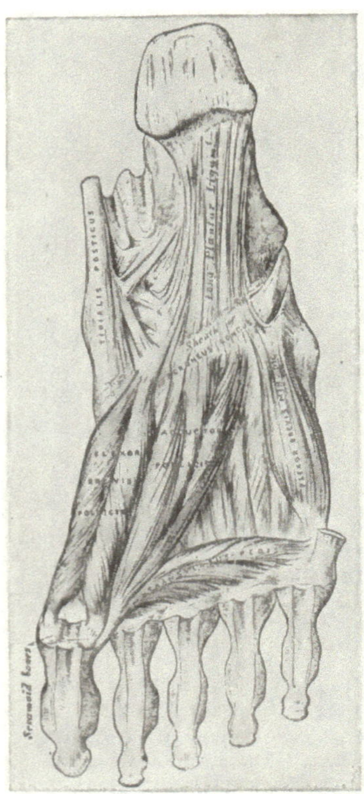

Muscles of the Sole of the Foot, third layer. (From Gray's Anatomy.)

Examination of normal foot prints shows (See Figs. 13, 14 and 15), as might be expected, that with increased pressure upon the foot there come into play accessory bearing surfaces on its sole. This is particularly evident in the appearance and increase in size of the inked spot, representing the second phalanx of the great toe, which is absent on the first of the above mentioned prints, made by the weight of the leg on the foot; in the second, partially fills the space between the balls of the foot and toe when the man marches under his own weight; and in the third almost completely fills this space when the man carries the military burden. The general broadening and lengthening of the foot under these diverse conditions of weight support is also apparent. These facts are important, since when troops are put into heavy marching order under burden, they bring into operation bearing areas of the feet

Fig. 13

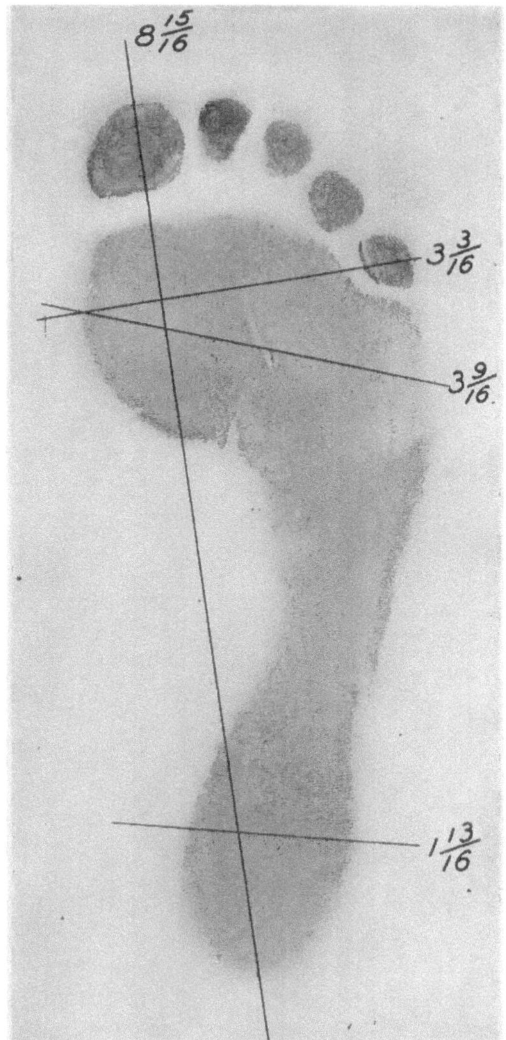

A normal foot print, taken with the soldier sitting. (Reduced.)

Fig. 14

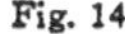

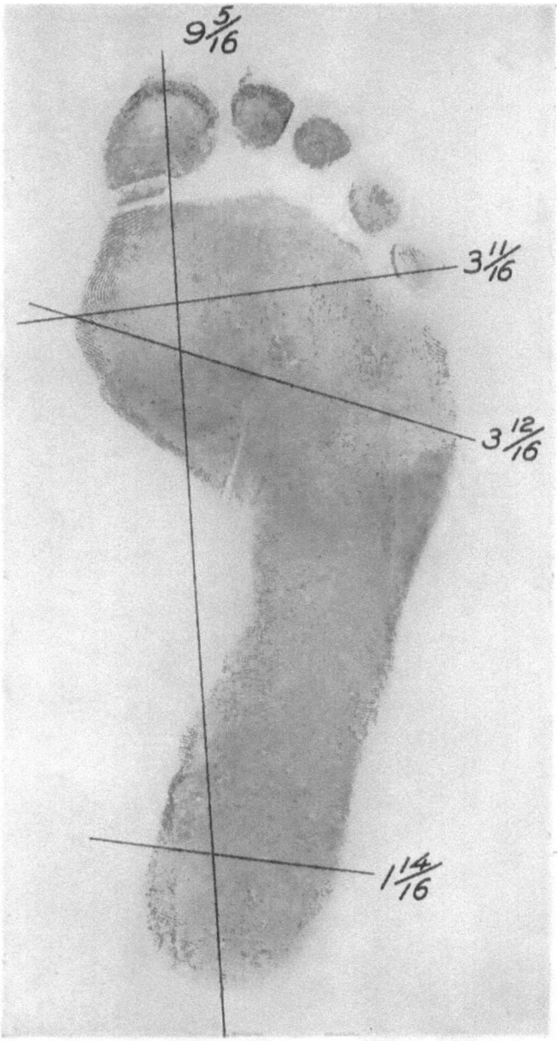

Foot print of the same foot shown in Fig. 13, but with the soldier walking without burden. (Reduced.)

Fig. 15

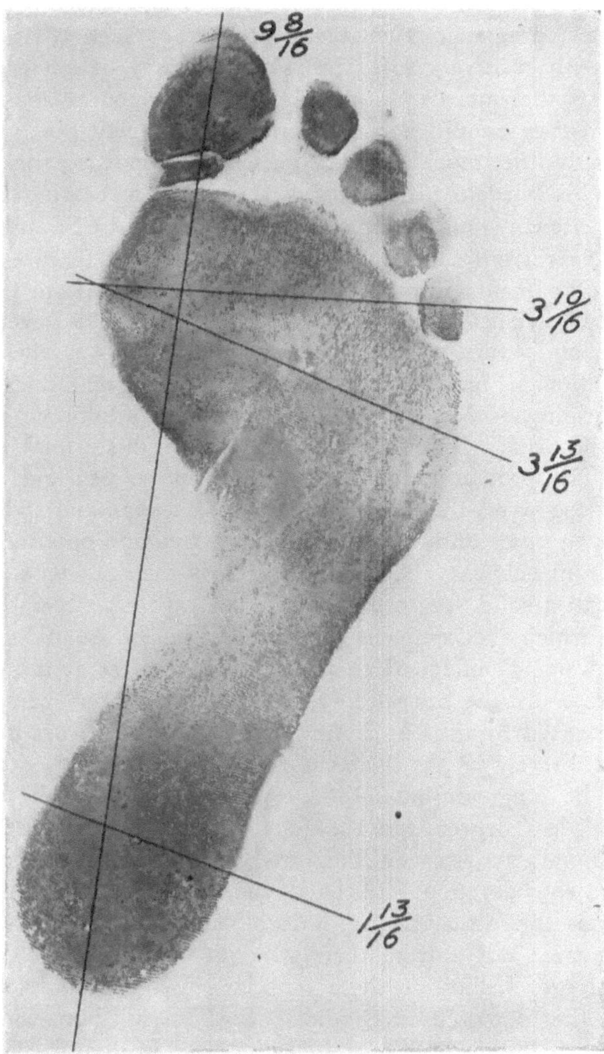

Foot print of the same foot shown in Figs. 13 and 14, but with soldier walking with a 40 lb. burden on his back. Compare with Figs. 13 and 14 to note increase in length and breadth. (Reduced.)

which have heretofore been largely unused and have thereby been protected against friction and pressure. Such areas are covered with relatively soft, thin skin and may be extremely sensitive at the outset of a march; but upon continuance of the march they should become hardened and play their part equally with other more toughened areas in supporting the soldier and his burden. Injury of such accessory bearing surfaces is quite common among soldiers at the outset of a march.

It is clear from a summary of the anatomical features of the bones, ligaments and muscles of the foot, that its most important part relates to the foot arch. The latter is a development in man to facilitate his characteristic walking in the upright position. Flat footed apes can walk no great distance in the upright position, and then only with the additional support of the arms. Flat footed men are notoriously unable to march. The foot arch has been shown not to be rigid, but to be a loose structure the bones of which wedge and tighten against each other under pressure from above and opposed by tension from below. The resulting arch is then not what engineers call a solid "segmental arch", but rather a "bowstring arch" in which the center is held up by tension on its ends. This "bowstring" effect of the muscles is greatest at the end of the step. If the pressure from above is greater than the tension exerted by the elastic muscles below, the excess pressure falls directly on the ligaments of the foot. If this excess pressure be long continued, the ligaments will stretch to a greater or less degree and the foot arch fall in proportion. But another factor, so well illustrated in Fig. 3, also has to be taken into consideration, and that is the size of the muscles located within the foot arch. With development of these muscles comes increase not only in their strength but in their bulk—and the larger bellies of these muscles, by more completely filling up the foot arch, mechanically hold up and buttress the latter against falling. Since muscles increase in the transverse diameter of their bellies on contraction—and as these foot muscles practically all run longitudinally—it becomes evident that the contraction of these muscles necessary to accomplish walking will at the same time serve not only to pull the ends of the foot arch together but to push up and support its sides and center. Too much importance therefore can not be placed in developing the foot muscles in preventing foot weakness, and such development is only brought about through their use, which in turn is only possible through proper foot-wear permitting of full function of the foot and the appropriate muscular action on which such function depends.

Fig. 11

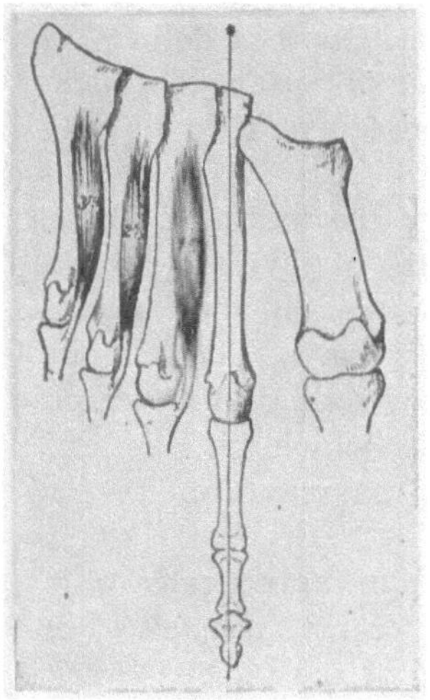

Muscles of the sole of the foot, fourth (plantar interosseous) layer. (From Gray's Anatomy.)

Fig. 12

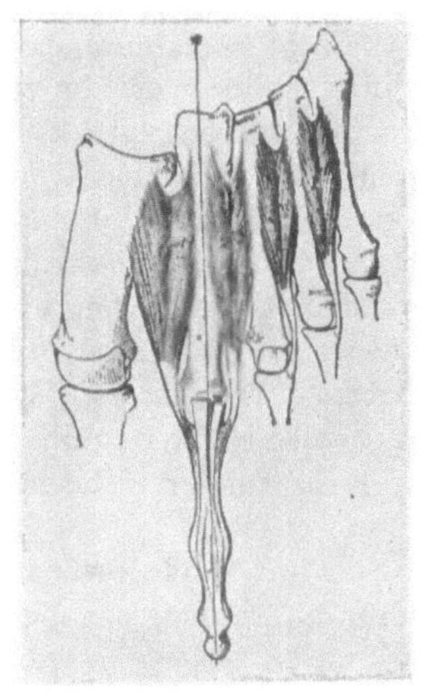

Muscles of the sole of the foot, fifth (interosseous) layer. (From Gray's Anatomy.)

Muscle tension and balance thus maintain the foot arch in its proper curvature. Where this is lost, the arch tends to flatten, with or without associated pain. But a foot of a type normally presenting a low arch may be quite as serviceable as if it were higher, since the muscle groups maintaining its integrity are satisfactorily performing all the work which is demanded of them. In stout, muscular feet the sole of the arch approaches nearer the ground than in unrelaxed arches with little muscular development; the difference is that with further loading of the individual with a burden, such as the military equipment, the first described arch remains about the same while the latter readily tends to break down.

Weakening of the foot muscles is one of the penalties of civilization, as walking is less and less a factor in locomotion, while primitive out-door peoples are more or less nomadic and their occupations are not sedentary. The introduction of railroads, street cars and automobiles, has materially interfered with foot development in many. And with lesser need for the use of the foot in walking, came the introduction of deforming and confining shoe types, by which the use of certain foot muscles was interfered with and their consequent atrophy and weakening was inevitable.

From consideration of the anatomy of the foot as a whole, it thus appears that the various structures of the foot form a whole which is both strong and supple; supple in the forward part and strong and massive in the hinder part. These points must not be forgotten, as they exert a controlling influence on the nature and shape of military footwear which must be provided for the soldier if he is to have a maximum ability for marching.

The perfect, undeformed foot is found practically only in children and among savage, non-shoe wearing peoples. See Figs. 16, 17, 18 and 19, in which the God of the famous Greek sculptor, the American child, and the head hunters of the Philippines present approximately the same foot type. As far as soldiers are concerned, the undeformed foot is a figment of the imagination; yet extreme cases of foot deformity, such as are common in civil life, are kept from admission to the military class through the requirements of the recruiting officer. However, in the great number of soldiers' feet examined by the Shoe Board, practically not one was free from some appreciable deformity or blemish. The production of foot injury begins early, and conditions become more serious, exaggerated and give less prospect of recovery with the passage of time. The condition is not so much produced by the mere fact of wearing shoes, as by the wearing of individual sets of shoes

Fig. 16

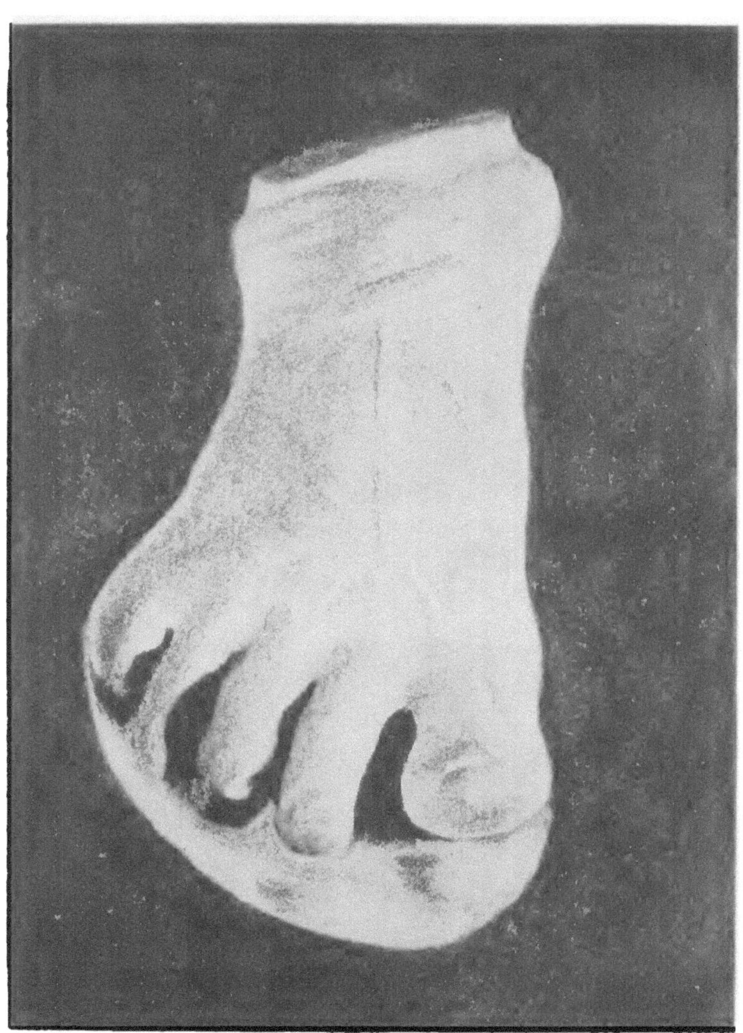

Foot of the "Flying Hermes" of Praxityles. Imprint of sandal strap, here not shown, appears on the foot. (From Weed.)

Fig. 17

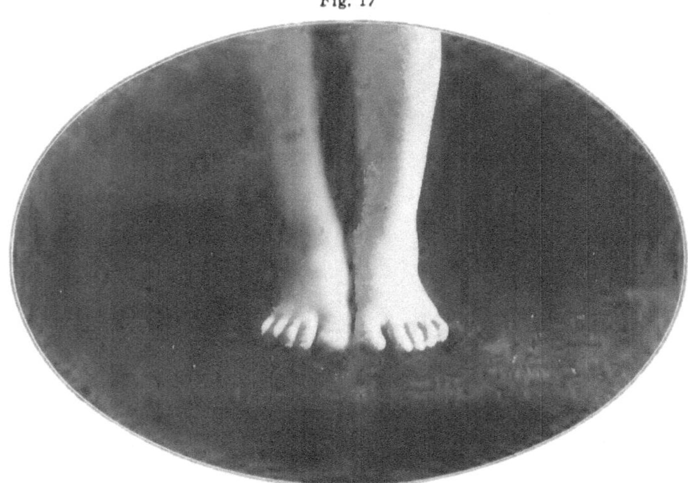

Feet of a four year old American child, undeformed by shoe wearing.

Fig. 18

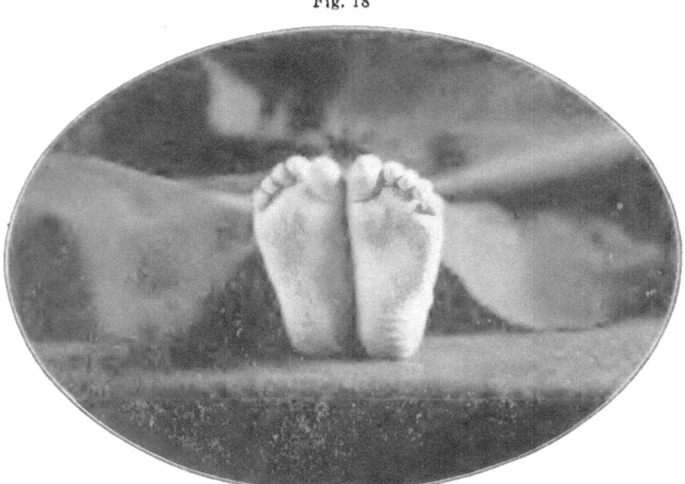

Feet same as those of Figure 17.

Fig. 19

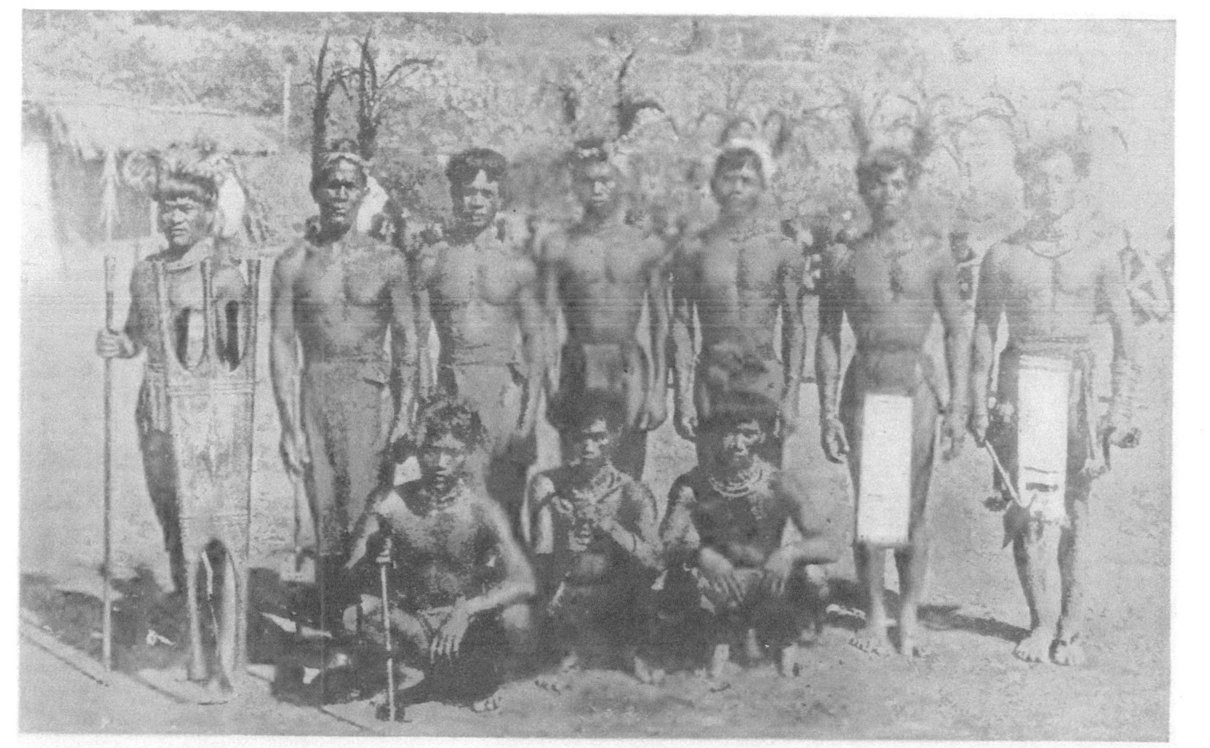

Bontoc Igorrotes of Lubuagan. Note the undeformed type of foot in the primitive savage, with spreading of the forefoot.

which do not fit. All shoes are not necessarily harmful to the feet, but careful attention to the character of the shoe and its subsequent appropriate fitting are both requisite in the avoidance of danger from this source.

The artificial results of deforming footwear, as seen for example in hallux valgus, are so common as to be accepted by many as the handiwork of nature. It is probable that a number of soldiers who regard the shoes issued by the government as "too broad", unconsciously express this erroneous idea.

It is quite apparent from the foregoing that the foot is not at all the rigid structure popularly supposed, to be carelessly jammed into any sort of container, irrespective of the size, shape, and character of the latter. On the contrary, it is seen to be a highly developed member of complex formation and intricate function, every factor of which needs thoughtful consideration in determining its proper covering.

Fig. 20

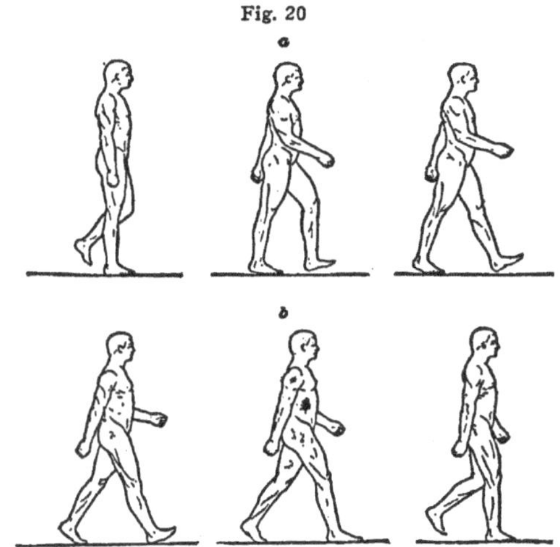

Military or Straight-leg Marching. (After Bradford.)

Having determined the anatomy of the foot, we may next briefly consider how the latter is used in marching (See Fig. 20). Shoes have their effect upon gait, and the shod man does not walk in the same manner as an unshod one.

Starting from a position, say, in which the sole of the right foot rests squarely on the ground and is practically supporting the entire body weight, the rear or left foot is just about to leave the ground against which its toes are pressed strongly by their flexor tendons. These toes are spread out and assist in maintaining equilibrium of the body, their bases are raised off the ground, and further contraction of their muscles causes the foot to rise until their tips rest against the ground and give a final push which sends the body further forward and destroys its equilibrium. This push need not be great, as the weight is now practically all supported by the right foot and balance is easily lost. To execute the last movement properly, it is clear that the shoe should be broad to allow for expansion, and its shape such that the great toe can stretch itself out directly forward in continuation of the long axis of the first metatarsal.

As this left foot leaves the ground the force of gravity, acting as a result of the loss of equilibrium in a forward direction, causes it to swing outward and brings it forward to a position under or slightly in front of the body without muscular exertion. From this point the leg is advanced through the distance required for the next step by the action of the extensor muscles and the straightening of the limb. At the same time the toes and front of the foot are pulled up by the muscles of the front of the leg. As the left foot strikes the ground, the body equilibrium temporarily lost is regained again through its support.

The heel strikes the ground first, with the toes pointed upward. The ankle joint is held firmly by the action of the muscular groups; the latter yielding as the center of gravity is advanced, and as more and more weight is thrown on this foot by propulsion from the right foot. The heel thus forms a fixed point with the ground, above which the body swings in a limited arc—the heel itself rotating until the toes are lowered and the foot rests squarely on the ground. In this last position the left foot is practically supporting all the body weight, which has now been transferred to it from the right foot.

The three chief points of support of the left foot are now the heel, and the heads of the first and fifth metatarsal bones. As in standing the foot arch bends slightly through its articulations yielding under the weight of the body and resumes its natural curve as soon as the foot is raised, so too this same limited joint motion of the arch occurs with every step in marching.

Fig. 21

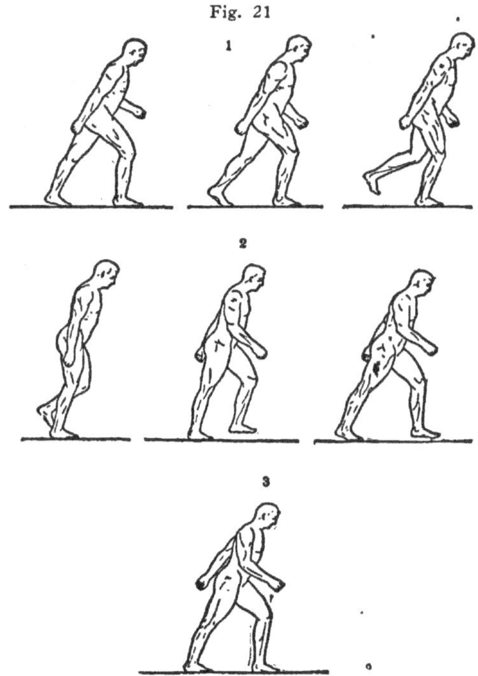

Flexion or Bent-knee Marching. (After Bradford.)

At this point, action of the muscles of the calf of the leg begins, supplements propulsion of the body from the right foot and lifts the left heel off the ground. In this position the point of support for the arch, and through it for the body weight, is in its anterior portion where the metatarsal bones rest upon the ground; the point of resistance, furnished by the ground and body weight, is on a level with the joint of the instep;

and the force is being applied to the heel bone, through the calf muscles.

In this position the body weight is being supported by the ball of the left foot, and is steadied and propelled forward by muscular action exerted through the right foot.

In the next stage, the intrinsic muscles of the sole of the left foot contract strongly to supplement the ligaments of the sole in preserving the foot arch, now under its maximum strain. At this point the toes leave the ground, the step is completed and a new cycle of foot and leg movement, as has just been described, begins. In the meantime the shoulders have been kept straight and the head and body are held erect. The knees are slightly flexed; while the free arm is allowed to swing naturally to better maintain the balance. This method of marching is not that voluntarily employed by the individual, who, when tired or not under restraint, tends to fall into the attitude and step of the flexion march (See Fig. 21) habitual to the bare footed races. In this latter step, the influence of gravity is greater and muscular effort less in moving the body forward, as the latter precedes rather than follows the advancing foot. The latter also strikes the ground more on the sole than the heel, and other differences in the step are apparent in comparison of the two illustrations.

Fig. 22

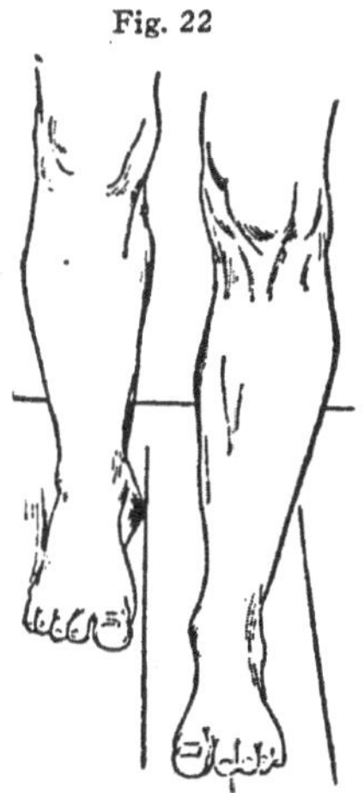

Illustrating the involuntary adduction of the fore-foot, due to the obliquity of the bearing surface of the metatarsus, in the proper attitude for walking. (Whitman).

In the ordinary step in marching, the toes should be directed well forward so that the thrust back in the foot, and especially in the great toe, shall be in the direction of its length rather than to a certain extent across it—since muscular action of the great toe is a potent agent in the propulsion of the body forward. (See Fig. 22).

If marching be done with an everted foot, the less the body is supported by the strong outer portion of the foot and the more the body weight is thrown upon the weak inner portion of the foot arch, not intended to support it. (See Fig. 23). In standing, moderate eversion of the feet better preserves equilibrium of the body by offering a broader basis of support—but in marching this is scarcely necessary, as with the rapid alteration of position the equilibrium lost at one step is instinctively regained at the next by alteration of balance or slight change of direction, as is the case in bicycle riding. Infantry Drill Regulations prescribe for the position of "attention" that the feet should be turned out at an angle of 45° ; but they make no mention as to the degree of eversion to be had in marching. If the toes are not deviated outward more than 25°, the weight begins to be thrown on the outer strong arch. Long standing is worse on the feet than marching, as there are no alternate periods of rest for the tired and relaxed muscles as is the case in walk-

Fig. 23

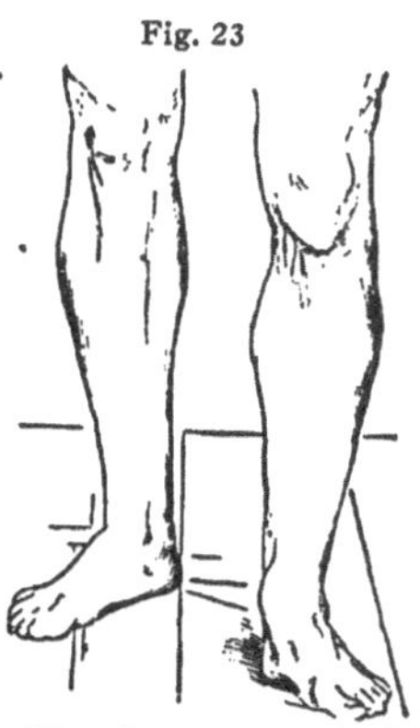

The improper attitude of outward rotation, in which there is disuse of the leverage function in standing and walking. (Whitman.)

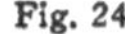

Fig. 24

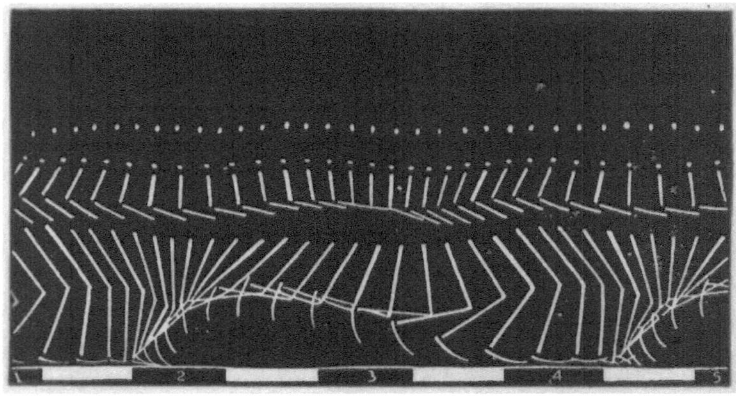

Positions of the Extremities of the Soldier During "Double Time." Photographs taken at the rate of sixty per second. (After Marey.)

ing. But care should be taken that the men should not be encouraged to walk "splay-footed", and any previous tendency that way should be rectified.

In marching in double time, the gait is quite different from that in ordinary marching (See Fig. 24). Here all the work is done by the ball and toes, the foot arch is under strong tension, and the heel only slightly touches the ground in preserving the balance. Running in narrow, pointed shoes at great speed, or for any considerable distance, is thus anatomically impossible.

CHAPTER III.

THE MILITARY SHOE.

All military authorities agree that a proper shoe for soldiers is a fundamental necessity in the accomplishment of military purposes. Marshal Niel stated that shoes for his infantry were of equal importance with mounts for his cavalry; while Wellington enumerated the three most essential parts of the soldier's outfit as a pair of good shoes, a second pair of good shoes, and a pair of half soles. And Marshal Bugeaud said: "Perhaps the two greatest problems of war are to find harness that will not injure horses and foot coverings that will not injure men."

There can be no question but that of all the protective coverings which the foot soldier wears, his shoes are by far the most important from a strategic standpoint; since upon their shape, durability, use and comfort of fit, pliancy and lightness depends his military efficiency. Next to his armament, the shoe is probably the most important item of the equipment of the soldier.

The construction of shoes for civilians is influenced almost wholly by considerations of fashion and style. These are irrational and are changed frequently in the financial interest of the shoe trade. The lasts are devised by persons grossly ignorant of, and quite indifferent to, the structure of the human foot and its physiological requirements as to covering. Shoes built upon them range through every degree of the bizarre and represent the most amazing conceptions of their originators as to the diverse shapes which the human foot should be forced to assume.

It is rare to find in civil life a shoe that even approaches the normal foot in shape and contour. Few manufacturers make them, as they are not salable to the general public, whose choice is swayed rather by considerations of fashion than comfort. For this reason, even the socalled orthopedic lasts do not accurately follow normal foot outlines under expansion but make certain concessions, as to narrowness and other matters, to popular ideas as to sightliness. Only in the case of the rare individual, who has from early life the sense and money to have his shoes built to order over plaster casts of his own foot, will suitably shaped and properly fitting shoes be found. The idea apparently dominating the construction of nearly all civilian shoes is that it is far better that foot wear should be novel in appearance rather than that it should be sensible in shape. A glance into the display window of the average shoe store will habitually show scores of varieties of shoes for adult males, of widely different appearance, not one of which even approaches correctness from an anatomical standpoint. Only for very young children can reasonably correct shoes be found. The reason for this is two fold. The shoe trade considers itself free from blame, as it is frankly in the business for profit, and is interested in giving the public what the latter thinks it wants. But this is only a half truth, for the nature of the foot wear which the shoe manufacturers themselves put out largely determines the public state of mind in this respect. On the other hand, all but a very few civilians are so influenced by the subtle suggestive influence of manufacturers' styles as largely to disregard matters of fit, shape and comfort, and tend to buy the enormities which the shoe manufacturers think it to be to their interest to put on the market. The very few who, despite such influences, would tend to prefer sensible shoes, receive little encouragement and frequently are quite unable to find in stock what they would like to purchase. A vicious circle is thus created, under which civilian shoe manufacturers and shoe wearers seem to vie with each other in injuring the feet. Add to this the firm resolve of nearly every civilian to crowd the foot into the narrowest and shortest shoe that it can be forced into without severe suffering, and the evil results to the foot are tremendously increased. The result is that practically every soldier in the army has had his feet more or less injured by the shoes he

Fig. 25

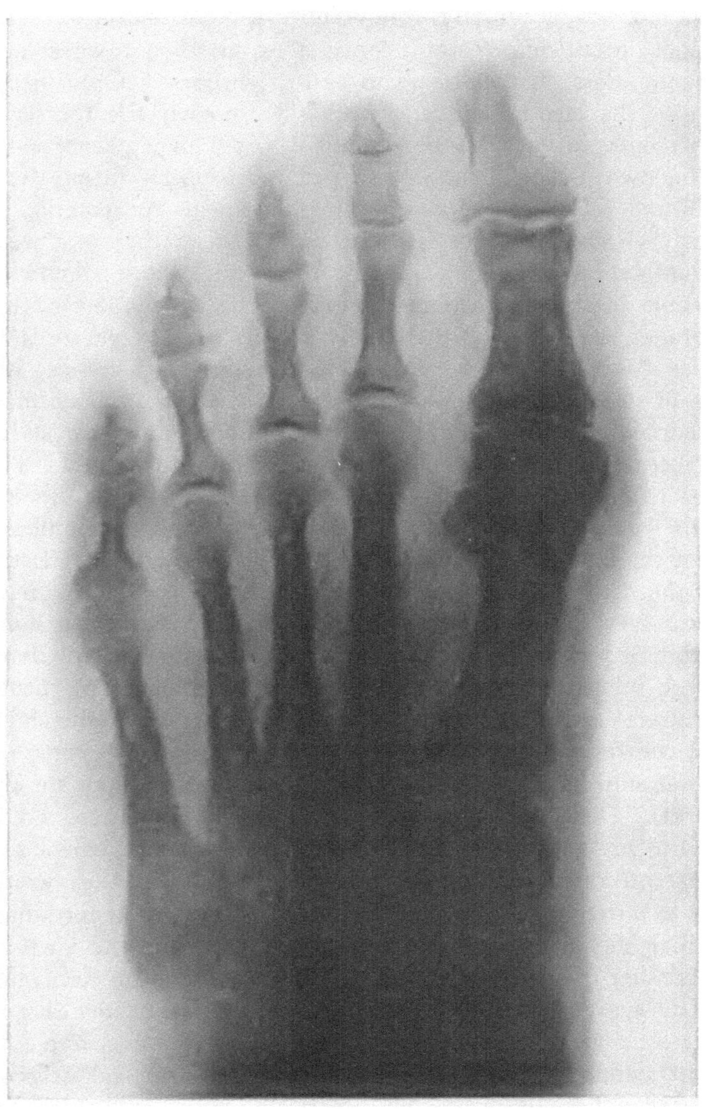

Foot of an officer bearing his weight on his naked foot.

Fig. 26

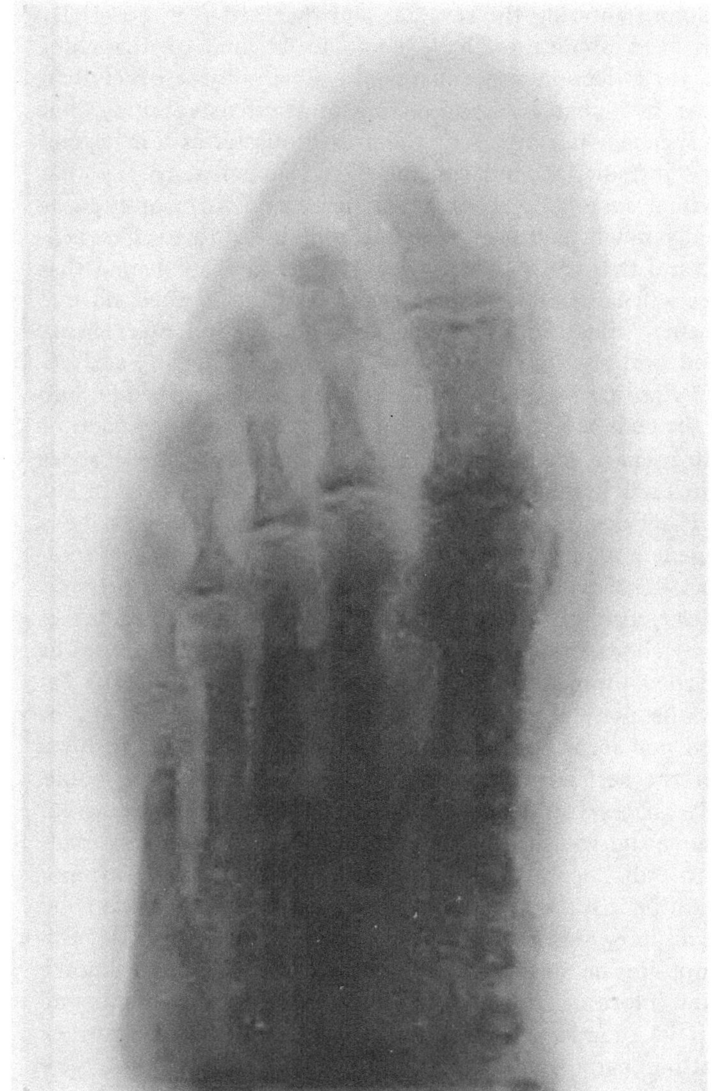

Same foot shown in Fig. 25 and under same body pressure, but in the civilian shoe which the officer wore on dress occasions. The foot is compressed over three quarters of an inch across the ball. (Reduction in size same as in Fig. 25).

wore before entering the service; and that bad feet, especially in city bred applicants, have come to be one of the chief causes for rejection for enlistment. The subject of civilian footwear is in itself an interesting and extensive study, but has no special connection with the present matter as it is beyond military jurisdiction and control. It is sufficient to say that the civilian shoe last, of whatever its special form or type, is habitually much narrower than the foot it is intended to represent, and that the vast majority of them are so shaped that the toes will be cramped together and bent out of their normal alignment. Illustrations of the foot before and after being crowded into such civilian shoes are given in Fig. 25 and 26. Also in Fig. 27, which well illustrates the abnormal shape into which the common style of civilian shoe compresses the foot.

But because such conditions as to foot-deforming shoes exist in civil life is no warrant for their continuance in the military service. The recruit, on enlistment, ceases to be a free agent and must wear as part of the uniform such footwear as the Government may, for its own interests, provide. The latter, also, can compel its contracting shoe manufacturers to supply shoes of specified shape, character and material. The whole shoe problem at once becomes simplified and thus becomes one merely of official jurisdiction and control—to be handled not according to individual whim or present fashion, but for the best advantage of the military service as a whole. Largely successful effort through supply of proper footwear to remove the foot blemishes incurred through mistakes made prior to enlistment, and to prevent the development of new ones, can be made immediately after entrance of the recruit into the military service. Nothing stands in the way of its efficient application except a too general lack of proper knowledge and interest in the subject, failure to appreciate the magnitude of its practical military importance, and the necessity of combatting erroneous preconceptions in the matter of shoe style and shoe fit on the part of not only of the recruit himself but too frequently in his company commander. Ignorance, indifference and passive opposition can do much to neutralize the best efforts in respect to improvement, and the special information required for their removal it is the purpose of this work to supply.

Good marching depends in its first cause upon a good shoe, so shaped and adapted to the foot as not to compress it, nor to unduly interfere with muscular action, nor to cause corns, bunions, ingrowing nails and other defects. No amount of liberality in the matter of supply, or the most scrupulous care in endeavoring to secure a fitting, can compensate for structural defect in a shoe supplied to troops. Given an inelastic container of bad shape, and the yielding tissues enclosed therein will be forced by pressure to assume a new, improper, and weaker foot form.

To meet the needs of the military service a special military shoe is required. No civilian shoe is adapted to the purpose. Civilian lasts as a whole are necessarily based in a general way upon the average civilian physical type engaged in various vocations of the average degree of civilian strenuosity. And in civil life, as already mentioned, average conditions tend materially to be against, rather than for, foot development. But the soldier at the very outset represents the physically elect of the class from which he comes and is better in this respect than its average; moreover, all his parts, including the feet, undergo development in strength and size under the active life, weight-carrying and systematized exercise which it falls upon him to perform after enlistment. That there is such a thing as a general military foot type, distinct from the average civilian foot, resulting from military conditions and training—just as civilian employments, as piano playing, shoe making and other callings bring about marked characteristic development of the hand—was advanced by the writer some years ago and later confirmed by the Shoe Board. To properly meet the special needs of the soldier, it thus became necessary to discard civilian lasts as not representing military foot types, remove the matter of footwear from the domain of speculation, and devise a new shoe adapted to military conditions, which should have as few faults and as many virtues as possible.

Fig. 27

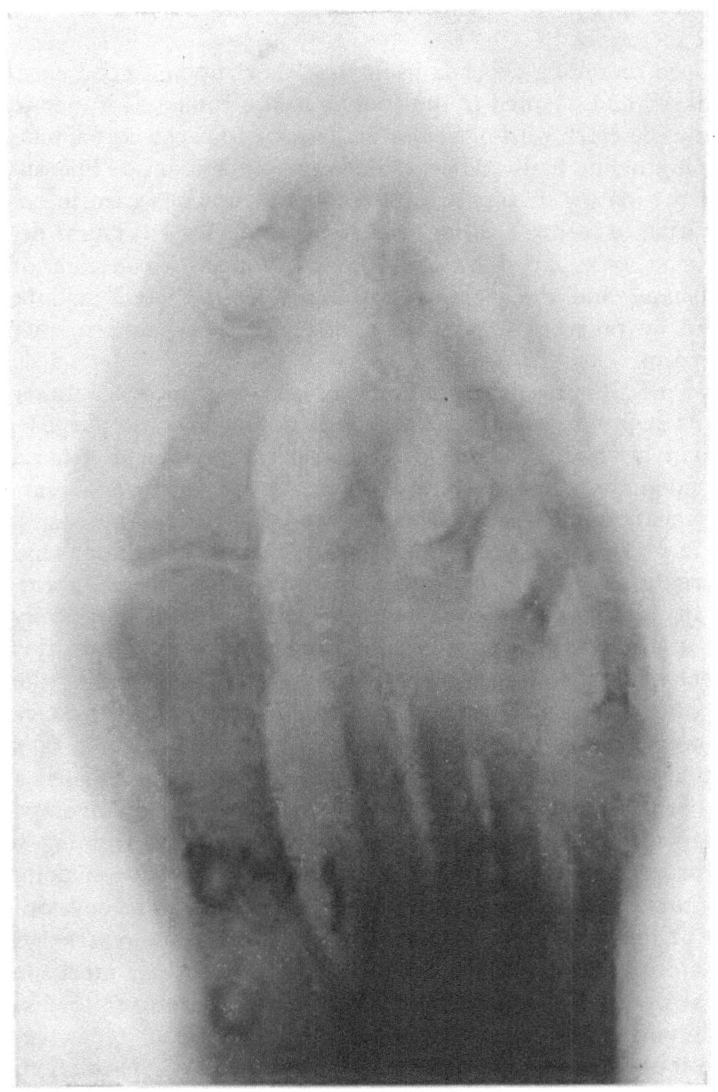

Foot of a soldier wearing a popular brand of civilian shoe.
Compare the appearance of this compressed foot with those shown in Figs. 16, 17, 18 and 19.

This has implied careful study not only in respect to footwear but of the special type of foot it was intended to cover; for the two are properly correlative and cannot be considered separately. The necessary work of investigation ultimately devolved upon the Shoe Board, which had various sessions during a period of four years. It is perhaps true that the whole subject of military footwear was gone into and considered more thoroughly by this board than was ever the case before. In this work the free use of the X-ray, in conclusively working out and visibly demonstrating foot relations under divers conditions—here systematically employed for the first time—proved very valuable.

There would seem to have been almost as many different ideas as to the proper type of footwear for military use as there are officers of the army. The great tendency among all is to generalize for the mass from the individual particular, and without mature reflection upon the very many weighty considerations necessarily involved. A very large number have some particular shoe which, found to be satisfactory for their own purposes as individuals under all or some conditions, they believe to be adapted for habitual use in the army as a whole. The Shoe Board has thus had recommended to it, as the ideal shoe for foot troops, almost every conceivable style and shape of footwear, beginning with a light, low, heelless shoe laced down over the ball, and through every intermediate type up to and including a heavy, double sole, hob-nailed, hunting boot, extending to above the knee.. Such widely divergent opinions are of course irreconcilable, and the board, while duly considering the merits of all such suggestions, ultimately found itself in the position of having to accept the great majority of them as representing merely the personal opinion of a single more or less competent observer. Of the latter, many were obviously biased, and approached the subject in a spirit of preference or prejudice. Many suggestions were also received from outside sources, more or less influenced by financial considerations in the hope of securing trade.

There are, however, certain fundamental requirements as

to construction, which probably all who have given even casual attention to the subject will agree should be incorporated in the military shoe. Any effort to work out such a shoe on a basis at once scientific and practical must give due consideration to them all, and perhaps the only ultimate difference of opinion in officers as a class will have to do with the proportionate degree in which each factor agreed upon as necessary should appear in the final result. The board entered upon its work in an absolutely unbiased frame of mind and uninfluenced by preconceptions; but soon came to the firm belief that the proper military shoe was a physiological one which must have as its basis the foot type found to exist in the average American soldier. And it accepted as conclusive that the military shoe must be so made that it will naturally tend to fit the foot of the average soldier, and not—conversely—that the foot of the recruit after enlistment must be made to conform to a foot covering built on arbitrary lines not in accordance with natural bulk and contours.

In view of the general ignorance and misapprehension respecting the anatomy of the human foot, the mechanics of marching, the results upon the feet of carrying a burden, the proper shape to be possessed by footwear, the requirements necessary to consider in fitting the shoe with suitable footwear, and other matters, it seemed desirable to take all these matters, hitherto largely in dispute, definitely and once for all out of the domain of idle speculation and mistaken hypothesis. This was done by the systematized use of the X-ray to show foot structure, and alteration in the anatomical relations of the foot, naked and in shoes of various sorts, under otherwise identical and perfectly comparable conditions.

It is believed that careful examination and proper interpretation of the radiographs appearing in this work will confirm the conclusions of the board as being founded upon fact rather than opinion, and will give a prompt and clear appreciation of many otherwise obscure matters relating to the soldier's foot and footwear.

The proper fundamental requirements which must enter

into every consideration of the shoe for the soldier were duly considered, incorporated into the final result, and here receive mention in the following discussion of the subject.

(a) A good military foot covering should be well joined, strong, substantial and solid, yet at the same time sufficiently flexible to permit of the natural functioning of the joints. It must be supple, so as to avoid the undue loss of necessary energy in overcoming resistance of the leather with each step—likewise to reduce the liability to blister and other injury. To attempt to use a stiff, unyielding shoe will result in the early falling out of a large proportion of its wearers. No better example of this can be found than the tremendous disability which occurred among the Germans as a result of the use of a shoe of this character. But on the other hand, the shoe can not be too soft and yielding, for the primary purpose of footwear is of course protection of the feet against injury. This includes protection against inequalities of the surface walked upon; the stones, sticks or other objects which may be inadvertently struck against; the keeping away of sand, mud, snow or other harmful substance; protection against cold in winter and heat in summer, also against dampness at all times.

(b) The shoe must be comfortable. This is an absolute essential to military footwear, for uncomfortable shoes will inevitably materially diminish the ability of troops to march. Shoe comfort depends, however, on the resultant of several factors, viz: a physiological shape, proper material, and suitable fitting. It also is affected not a little by foot condition. Detailed discussions of these matters appear elsewhere; but it may here be mentioned that to the best of its ability, nothing has been left undone by the Shoe Board, from the standpoint of scientific theory as fortified by the results of experimental trial, which could in any way enhance the comfort of the military shoe for the soldier class as a whole.

(c) The shoe must be durable. The soldier's foot covering is subjected to extreme tests of durability in the field, being necessarily worn through dust, mud and water, or over sand or rocks as the case may be. Questions of continued adequacy of foot protection and of difficulties of resupply in campaign require that wearing qualities shall be the best. With shoe-wearing peoples, when shoes wear out marching capacity practically ceases. To ensure that only material having the very best wearing qualities shall be used in manufacture of the military shoe is thus true military economy. The original virtues of the material may be long retained by proper care. The main wear of course falls on the soles. These are now made as thick and strong as the choicest cuts of the thickest sides of leather will permit. They cannot be increased in durability except by the use of double soles, which latter are unnecessarily heavy, stiff and hard on the feet.

As the soles wear thin to a point where inequalities of the ground hurt the feet, provision should be at hand, in the form of half soles, to be readily attached as required, to secure further use of the shoe without discarding the still good uppers.

(d) The shoe should be as simple and neat as possible. A plain finish is desirable. Box toes improve the appearance of the shoe, but they are made of sole leather which is moulded into shape when wet, and this shape is retained only so long as they are not again saturated with water. They have the serious defect, when wet and drying off the feet, of warping, shrinking and curving down at the posterior margin in the formation of a stiff, sharp edge which presses down over the toes and is practically certain to cause foot injury on marching. Where the soldier comes into camp wet and tired, he is apt to throw his shoes aside without thought of their condition in the morning. To eliminate the source of danger which box toes thus offer, they have been left off the military shoe, whose double thickness of leather over the toes is believed to give the latter all necessary protection.

Neatness in appearance is desirable in so long as it does not interfere with efficiency. One advantage in this respect in not having the shoes oil-stuffed before issue is that they can be highly polished for inspection and special formations, such as guard mount. While it has the essential advantage of being built on a physiological foot-form, the new shoe appears much less clumsy and cumbersome than most of the more or less rational army shoes which were its predecessors.

(e) The foot covering should be as light in weight as is compatible with serviceability. This point has been constantly borne in mind; it being appreciated that even a small additional weight on the foot will very materially interfere with marching capacity. The much greater effort required for marching under the drag of even a small amount of mud adhering to the shoe is commonly known. That an extra amount of weight on the foot may materially alter the gait is well understood by all horseman and applies equally to human beings. In working out the new shoe, it was made to weigh as little as would be compatible with durability. Every particle of material that could be spared was cut away. The result is a shoe which weighs only about two and one-half ounces more than the former garrison tan shoe, and can in no way be regarded as heavy or cumbersome for military use. It is of much less weight than are certain types of footwear more or less commonly used by pedestrians, mountain climbers, hunters, prospectors, farmers and others whose work or recreation requires much walking in the open. It will at first appear slightly heavy, however, to recruits previously accustomed to wear civilian shoes of the ordinary light civilian type; but this impression of somewhat greater heaviness disappears in a few days when the foot and leg muscles develop and strengthen to accommodate themselves to changed conditions of weight bearing.

(f) The shoe must be made in such a way that the soldier can easily put it on and take it off. This is a practical point, the need for which is obvious to all conversant with the military service. To facilitate it, the shoe must be capable of opening widely, and the number of holes for lacing reduced to the lowest limit compatible with the holding of the shoe firmly around the ankle and over the instep. The new military shoe has a wide half-bellows tongue and but six eyelets on a side.

from only one or two of which the lace need be withdrawn in order to readily put the foot in or take it out.

(g) The material of which the shoe is made, and the special treatment of the former, must be such as will facilitate evaporation of moisture from within, yet not to a degree by which the absorption of moisture from without is unduly favored. It must have pores through which a certain amount of air can pass; also qualities of capillarity by which moisture is transferred from a damp sock to the outside of the leather where evaporation is rapid. This is very important, since otherwise the retained perspiration will keep the feet damp all the time, while interference with evaporation will make them uncomfortably hot in warm weather. Under the combination of dampness and heat, the superficial layer of the skin becomes moisture-soaked, soft, tender, and apt to break down in the formation of blisters and abrasions. Yet on the other hand, the shoe material should be sufficiently water-repellant to keep the feet reasonably dry under ordinary conditions of rain and dew. Such material can be secured; it is true that it is not perfect for any extreme condition, but best meets the needs of the every day and average conditions upon which the requirements of the soldier's shoe must be based. If it is desired for climatic or seasonal changes to have the soldier's shoe more waterproof, this condition can be produced as required quite as well by the soldier himself without the necessity of having it done in advance. For these reasons, in developing the recent military shoe, it was thought preferable to use leather of vegetable tan rather than chrome tan, since in the latter the pores of the leather are largely filled up with an impermeable deposit. For similar reasons, leather "stuffed" or saturated with oil was not used. Shoes can be made quite water repellant with a little oil but without saturation by it; on the same principle that the almost imperceptible greasiness of a duck's feather causes water falling on its back to break into minute droplets which roll off without wetting. And shoes thus lightly oiled will still permit of passage of moisture laden air as vapor through the leather, while holding out water in bulk unless under considerable pressure sufficient to force it in through the pores of the material.

(h) The material or leather of the shoe upper must not be hard; otherwise it will cause blisters, callouses and corns. The "brogans" formerly issued in our service, and the footwear of various foreign armies, have this defect. Apparent hardness may be reduced by the addition of a lining to the shoe, but the usual effort of the soldier to secure this end consists in getting very roomy shoes so that thick, heavy socks may be used as a cushion to diminish the dangers of friction and impact. In the present shoe, the leather selected for the upper is as soft and yielding as is compatible with sufficient thickness and durability.

(i) The cost of the military shoe is a consideration quite secondary to the one of efficiency. The footwear of the soldier, as elsewhere stated, is the very last article of his apparel upon which to practice economy. Shoes are properly to be regarded as much more than mere clothing; they are the agent on which the mobility of infantry depends and the accomplishment of tactical purposes is possible. In the end, the best shoe is by far the cheapest, and the economic loss alone—disregarding tactical considerations—resulting from the disability of even a few men by poor shoes, after a large amount of money, time and effort has been expended to prepare them for the emergency in which they are found wanting, is far greater than any saving which could be made on many thousands of pairs of shoes. However, this does not mean that a proper military shoe is necessarily an unduly expensive one. It costs no more to make a shoe on a good last than on a bad one and the factor of labor is approximately the same. Only in cost of material is there any material difference, and this is more than compensated for by the greater life of the high class shoe. True shoe cost is not a matter of original outlay, but has relation to the average number of day's wear which can ultimately be obtained from the article in question. The military shoe recently designed costs no more than military shoes of the past.

(j) By reason of the relations which must exist between the different sizes and widths of the general military type of foot which it is intended to cover, a sufficient number of sizes as to length, and letters as to width, must be provided in order that the foot of every soldier may find a shoe of dimensions to properly cover it. This point is taken up in some detail under the subject of fitting of the shoe. It is sufficient here to say that the Shoe Board has recommended that shoes be made in fifteen sizes and half sizes, and that each of these be made in six widths, giving a total of ninety varieties of shoes from which to make selection.

(k) The shoe should be perfectly smooth in the interior, especially the insole, the part surrounding the heel and the uppers over the fore foot. This is largely a matter of proper manufacture, to be enforced by vigorous inspection before acceptance from the contractor by the Government. Seams must be sewed smoothly, and any rough edges so apt to hurt the foot must be cut away. There must be no seam at the rear of the heel to thus create more or less roughness over an area particularly liable to injury; rather there should be a heel piece with the seam at the side. The insole must be cut accurately to proper size so that it will fit the shoe—if too small, it leaves a depressed space between its edges and the margins of the foot, into which the latter overlap to their injury; if too large, its edges will tend to curve up on drying after wetting or constant exposure to sweat; and inequality of the other type, but equally hurtful to the foot, is thus produced. The upper surface of the heel is usually rough from nails which have been pounded back and clinched into position. To cover its inequalities, a sock piece of sheepskin or calfskin is usually glued into position over it. This, if badly done with inferior adhesive material, will probably result in the leather piece wrinkling and ultimately working loose under the combined influence of moisture and friction, the effect of which is to create an uneven bearing surface for the heel which in marching will probably cause its injury. The only material suitable to fasten this heel-piece in position is the best quality of rubber cement, which will resist the disturbing agencies mentioned. The drill lining of the shoes, if put in position by the common careless method of manufactures, will wrinkle and fold over the toes, causing serious foot trouble. This drill lining is usually tacked on over the last, wet like the leather with which it is used. But leather expands and stretches better to fit the last while wet, while wetted canvas shrinks, as is evidenced by tentage in a rain storm. On the drying of both, the leather retains its new shape and size, while the contained canvas relaxes and enlarges and becomes redundant and wrinkled for the space it is intended to cover. The remedy is, in making the shoe, to stretch the canvas lining over the last dry, and to fasten it smoothly to the leather over the toes by a thin layer of rubber cement. All these points have been duly acted upon in connection with the manufacture of the new shoe.

(1) The heel should be broad, flat, long and solid. When the soldier stands erect, the heel is the chief point of support of the weight of the body and burden, with the bases of the great and little toes forming accessory points of support. The latter check any tendency to rotation of the heel, resulting from shifting of the body weight. A large, broad heel affords a better bearing surface and grip on the ground, and by so much reduces the muscular tension required to maintain equilibrium of the body in standing and walking. Its surface should be flat; otherwise the sole of the foot will be inclined at more or less of an angle away from its proper horizontal plane, and this abnormal position requires constant muscular effort to counteract it, with interference with marching and liability to sprain. In persons who toe out, as in most shoe wearing peoples, the outer margin of the heel strikes the ground first and forms the fixed point over which the weight of the body and burden is supported. The result is that this outer edge of the heel tends rapidly to wear under the combined influence of much weight and friction acting on a small area. To avoid this wearing and alteration of foot plane as much as possible, the outer half of the heel is heavily reinforced with iron nails.

The heel must be low, since raising it will throw the center of gravity of the body forward on the foot, thereby bringing an undue amount of pressure on the foot arch which was never intended by nature to support it and may yield and flatten under the strain. Also it will force the foot forward in the shoe, bring undue strain across the instep, and, unless the shoe is very long, jam the toes to their injury against the front of the shoe. Finally, the plane of the lower face of the heel should correspond with that of the sole, so as to give the most secure bearing surface on standing. All these points have been considered in devising the new military shoe.

(m) The inside of the shoe over the heel should not be too wide. This is necessary in order that there may not be slippage of the heel of the foot from side to side within the shoe, with resulting heel blisters. The inside width of the shoe in this region should be such as will hold the foot comfortably, and under the pressure of the body weight and burden will be filled by the flattened heel without compressing the latter. Reduction in heel width was made in the new shoe.

(n) The posterior wall of the shoe should be curved so as to embrace the natural curvature of the heel. This is necessary to hold the rear part of the foot in position and reduce friction on the heel by preventing it from slipping up and down and chafing against the shoe in marching. This important point has been overlooked in some of the military shoes of the past—notably the old "brogan" and the more recent high marching shoe (See Fig. 36)—but has been duly considered in the latest pattern of foot wear.

(o) The shoe should not support the arch of the foot in the sense of lifting it up or buttressing it from below. This fact is opposed to common belief, but the latter is based on lack of knowledge of the anatomy of the foot and misconception as to its function. Rigid support of this region weakens its intrinsic muscles by favoring their non-use, and thus tends to directly cause the condition of flat-footedness which it is attempted to avoid. Barefoot peoples have no such arch support and flat feet are practically unknown among them. As this matter of arch support is fully discussed later under the subject of flat-feet, it needs no further consideration here. In the new shoe, the purpose is to have the leather accurately follow the outlines of the average soldier's foot arch, but without compressing the sole muscles to such an extent that their function will be interfered with and their development and strengthening be impaired. Every structure of the foot concerned in marching should be left free to function to the best anatomical and mechanical advantage. For this reason, the new shoe has no metal shank as stiffening under the foot arch.

(p) The sole should be sufficiently thick to prevent the foot from being injured by inequality in the ground. But if too thick, planter flexion of the foot is lost and dorsi-flexion is much reduced. The foot is thus reduced to the condition of a solid block, hinging at the ankle and simply furnishing a solid support to the leg. Moreover, with thick soles, the leverage function of the great toe is interfered with, and the push of the foot is across the whole breadth of the sole at the metatarso—phalangeal joint. The sole of the present shoe is as thick as can be made of one thickness of the best sole leather; to make it of two thicknesses would add slightly to protection and subtract greatly from foot power and comfort.

(q) The sole should be flat across, to furnish a level surface for the foot and a more secure hold upon the ground in steadying the body in standing and marching. It should have a slight upward curve at its forward end to prevent the toe catching in unevenly raised places on the walking surface, and to permit of accomplishing the heel-and-toe-walking of the marching step. But this curve or "spring" should not be too great or the toes will be placed, as a result of insufficient leather in the upper, in a permanent condition of hyper-extension which interferes with walking and stability in standing. Some officers have advised a very considerable "spring" to the shoe, apparently under the idea that walking is a kind of rolling or rocking-chair-motion—which of course is not at all the case.

In marching with the naked foot, all parts of its bearing surfaces are in simultaneous contact with the surface beneath at one period of the accomplishment of the step. In other words, all anterior parts of the toes are in strong propulsive contact with this surface before the heel leaves it. Too much "spring" in the sole would mechanically interfere with the accomplishment of this relation. Sufficient curvature or "spring" of the sole, to better suit the peculiarities of individual feet, will in any case be soon developed by sufficient use.

(r) There must be plenty of room across the ball of the foot, so that there shall be no constriction of the weight bearing foot at that point. Under continued marching, the foot is given to flattening somewhat more—particularly at the end of a march when the muscles are tired and tend to relax—than it did at the trial fitting; likewise, the foot will swell from pressure interfering with the circulation. Moreover, the metatarsal bones tend to separate more widely from each other in marching. And as the points of support of the foot may practically be regarded as the legs of a tripod passing through the heel and the fronts of the metatarsal bones of the great and little toes, it is evident that the more the legs of this tripod can diverge the greater will be its stability as a whole. Also if the ball of the foot be regarded as a fulcrum, the greater the width of this fulcrum the greater the lateral stability of the superimposed body. Breadth across the ball is a characteristic feature of the new shoe.

(s) The toe cap must be high, so as to avoid any hurtful pressure on the toes below. It must also rise abruptly from the front of the shoe, without forming an acute angle into which the front of the toes may be wedged in walking. Lowness over the toes was a most serious defect in the old marching shoe, resulting in a vast number of blisters on top of the toes and not infrequently in loss of toe nails, usually of the great toe, which from its greater height received most of the pressure. This fault has been remedied in the new shoe of the Shoe Board, which is three-sixteenths of an inch higher over the toes than its predecessor. Three-sixteenths of an inch may not seem a great increase, but as it has been added over the entire toe region, which measures approximately two and one-half inches in the shoe across the toe from sole to sole, it has added approximately one-half of a square inch to the sectional area enclosed by the shoe in this region. This increased height might not be enough if the shoe were a rigid container or had a box toe; it is, however, a liberal increase when it is remembered that the toe cap is soft, pliable and readily alters in shape, and unnecessary excess of leather over the smaller toes is diminished and flattened down under any upward pressure of the great toe with compensating increase in material and height over the latter. As the breadth of the great toe is only about an inch, and the total addition of leather in the toe cap is nearly all available to increase the height of the shoe above it, it is evident that the recent increase in height of the toe cap permits of its elevation over the great toe from a third to half an inch greater than formerly. This increase in possible height over the great toe is believed to be quite sufficient to meet the needs of theory, and has been so demonstrated in practice.

(t) The material of the quarters must be pliable. This is necessary so that the shoe may readily yield, without the formation of hard creases and ridges, to the movements of the ankle joint. Stiffness of leather in the quarters would seriously interfere with marching and promptly cause painful abrasions around the ankle. Nor must the quarters be cut any higher than necessary, as adding materially to the weight and cumbrousness of the shoe without giving any corresponding advantage. So long as a legging is worn, the military footwear should be a shoe, and to make it higher than the new military shoe would bring it into the boot or half-boot class. The latter has been tried out in our service and found undesirable. For the vast majority of conditions encountered by the soldier, the height of a shoe reaching a little above the ankle is quite satisfactory.

(u) There should be no stiff or excessive leather, or rows of stitching, so located as to be immediately over any of the extensor tendons of the toes, which lie close to the surface over the instep. This particularly applies to the extensor tendon of the great toe. These hard, rough areas tend to compress and injure the tendons sliding beneath them and cause pain and irritation. In the new military shoe, this matter has received careful attention, and areas of stitching have been decreased in size and the seams of the quarters brought lower on the sides of the foot. This also permits of a little more stretching of the leather over the instep, which is desirable in many cases.

(v) The tongue should be as small as possible to prevent bunching and wrinkling under the laces, with injury to the instep. In the new shoe, the tongue has been reduced in thickness as much as practicable. The full bellows has been changed to half-bellows, as the excess of leather of the former caused much discomfort, made it more difficult to get in and out of the shoe, interfered somewhat with evaporation of perspiration and gave, in practice, no appreciable increase of protection of the foot against water, mud and dust.

(w) The front of the quarters must be sufficiently cut away so that the rows of eyelets may be well separated in order to provide elasticity in the fitting of different heights of instep. It is not at all essential to foot comfort that the quarters should nearly meet when the shoe is laced up, since the half-bellows tongue closes the front of the shoe against sand and dirt. But it is very essential that the margin of the quarters shall be far enough apart to permit of snug lacing on feet with low insteps, else slippage of the shoe on the foot is certain to result.

(x) Eyelets, and not hooks, must be used for the laces. The latter are not held with certainty by hooks, and frequent readjustments on the march may thus be necessary. Moreover, hooks bend, break and rapidly wear out the shoe laces, while causing undesirable rubbing and wear on the lower part of the legging. The substitution of hooks only saves time in fastening and unfastening the shoe where many eyelets are concerned—but time would be lost if the military shoe, with its few eyelets, had hooks instead; for unfastening the lacing with the latter loosens it completely as far as they extend.

(y) The shoe must have such a shape that it will not contain any useless dead space, since these require extra material as a covering, which would cause unnecessary weight and encumbrance to the foot. In the old marching shoe, considerable excess space of this nature was present in front of the smaller toes. The Shoe Board found by use of the X-ray and by experimental marching that this space could be considerably reduced and a little material cut away from this region without the slightest danger of the smaller toes striking against the front of the toe cap. Compare, in this connection, Figs. 33 and 34. This change also improved the appearance of the shoe by giving it a tapering effect in the direction of the great toe. This cutting away of the material was gradual and began about one inch behind the toe cap, or about opposite the end of the little toe, curving in toward the great toe with a maximum width of approximately one quarter of an inch.

(z) The shoe must also have such a shape as to permit of the great toe returning toward its proper alignment to the degree which the average age and ordinary foot deformity of the soldier class would warrant reasonable expectation. That none of the shoes previously supplied in our army were properly shaped in this respect was visibly demonstrated by many radiographs taken by the Shoe Board, as well as by the marked hallux valgus and blisters and ingrowing nails common among soldiers and indicating pressure against the inner aspect of the great toe. To remedy this fault, a suitable amount of additional space internal to the great toe was needed, but the amount so required was not capable of mathematical demonstration. It was not difficult to formulate such internal lines for an ideal last, since in this case a straight line from the inner margin of the heel would fall along the inner margin of the sole. It was possible to measure a number of feet, and determine thereupon the degree of deviation of the average toe; but such results would be inconclusive, since they would not

Fig. 28

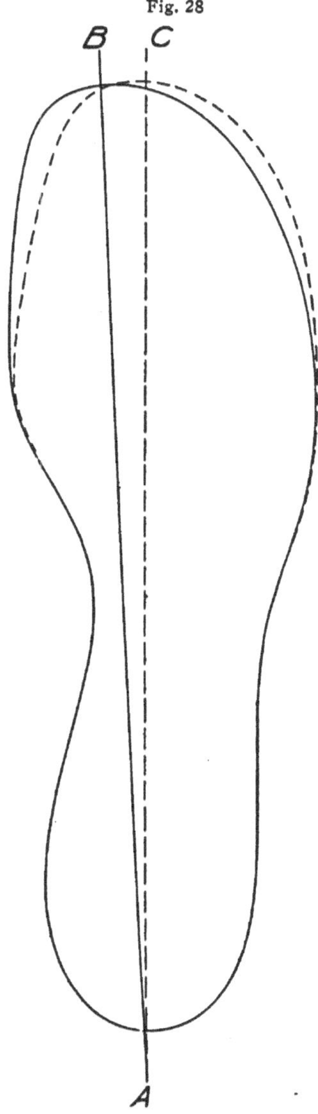

Tracings of new (solid line) and old (dotted line) insoles. (reduced.)

take into consideration the amount of correction in the present faulty alignment of the great toe which might be expected to ultimately occur in the foot of the average soldier if enclosed in a shoe of physiological shape and sufficient width. The latter was a subject never before studied and of which nothing was known; nor could it be scientifically so studied except by an extensive series of experiments based on suitable shoes and covering a long period of time in a class of soldiers of various ages. But the Shoe Board, in its study of thousands of feet, had naturally arrived at fairly positive conclusions of its own in respect to the average amount of foot deformity present in American soldiers, and the extent to which its natural correction under favorable conditions might reasonably be anticipated.

It took into consideration the fact that the average soldier has deformed feet as a result of habitual use of improper shoes since childhood, and has reached an age in life when development is completed and any alteration in the relations of the skeleton of the foot—for example, in the throwing of the great toe out of its proper axis, as in hallux valgus—tends to become in considerable part permanent. The best to be expected in the shape of the practical military shoe are therefore not the ideal lines which would properly be found in a covering for ideal feet; but rather sufficient provision that its shape shall not only no longer tend to increase or perpetuate the deviation but shall permit of such reasonable tendency to return of the toe to normal alignment as may fairly be expected of the average soldier.

With this standard in mind, the board proceeded to add more space to the inner aspect of the great toe, beginning at its metatarso-phalangeal joint and gradually increasing to a maximum width of something over a quarter of an inch opposite the nail of the great toe. (Compare Figs. 33 and 34). Though this does not seem a great increase, in practice it amounts to straightening the inner lines of the shoe and giving additional space to an extent as great as the average soldier's foot can probably ever utilize. This is borne out by extensive radiographic study of soldiers' feet in shoes so modified, and determining by touch the amount of excess space which the deviated great toe at first did not utilize.

Fig. 29

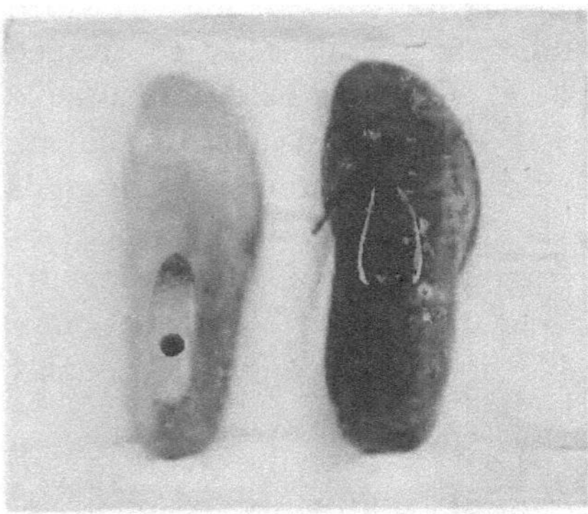

The new military last and shoe.

The shoe constructed on this last, as just indicated, will have an inward curve in front of the shank, which produces an apparent slight adduction—or position of greater strength—of the foot and allows it to point more to the front in walking. This tends to throw the weight off the foot-arch, and upon the outer and stronger part of the foot where it belongs. This twist of the forepart of the shoe is maintained by the shape and thickness of the sole, reinforced toward the rear by a stout leather shank which holds the sole rigid from side to side while permitting its necessary bending in other directions. This bend or twist in front of the shank of the shoe exists in a degree which is only physiological; in fact, it was based on the conception of the Shoe Board on this point as a result of its large number of foot examinations. The purpose is to have the foot rest on the shoe sole in its natural position, and there is no pressure on the little toe calculated to turn the fore-foot inward away from its proper alignment. And it has been found that the average military foot, placed within the outline tracing of the sole of a new style military shoe which fits it, bears a very close relation in its horizontal plane to such an outline. The sole of the new shoe is thus physiological in shape. The very marked difference in shape of sole between the new military shoe and the marching shoe which preceded it, and the difference in position of the feet which would be within them, is shown in the accompanying illustration (Fig. 28), in which tracings are made of the respective insoles of the same size shoes after accurately fitting their heel and shank portions to the same areas. Lines are drawn from the common point A at middle of rear of heel to the furthest point at the front of each toe—the solid line AB representing the longitudinal axis of the new shoe of the Shoe Board, while the broken line AC represents that of the preceding marching shoe. It was determined that the apparently slight changes made by the Shoe Board in the shape of the sole have resulted in the shifting of the axis of the foot by approximately three quarters of an inch nearer normal at the toe. This change should be of very considerable assistance to marching, prevent the development of toe deformity and do much to ultimately rectify such of the latter as has occurred in other than very old cases.

Fig. 30

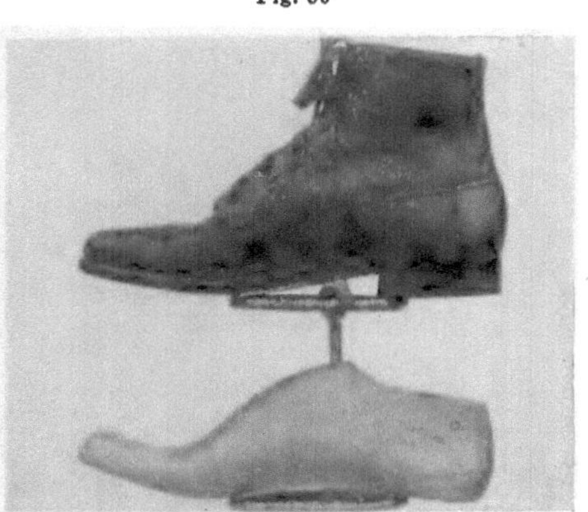

The new military last and shoe.

The new military shoe and the last on which it is made are illustrated in Figs. 29 and 30.

The shoe last and shoe finally evolved as a result of study of the foregoing requirements is not based on preference, prejudice or preconception. In its outlines, prevailing styles embodying the temporary whims of fashion were not taken into account. It is believed, however, that it closely coordinates with the shape, volume and physiological functions of the foot. This seems apparent from a comparison of Figs. 31, 32, 33 and 34, in which the same soldier's foot, of a good type, is successively shown radiographed, under the identical conditions of pressure resulting from carrying a 40 lb. burden, with naked foot, with foot in the garrison tan shoe, in the old marching shoe, and in the new military shoe. It will

Fig. 31

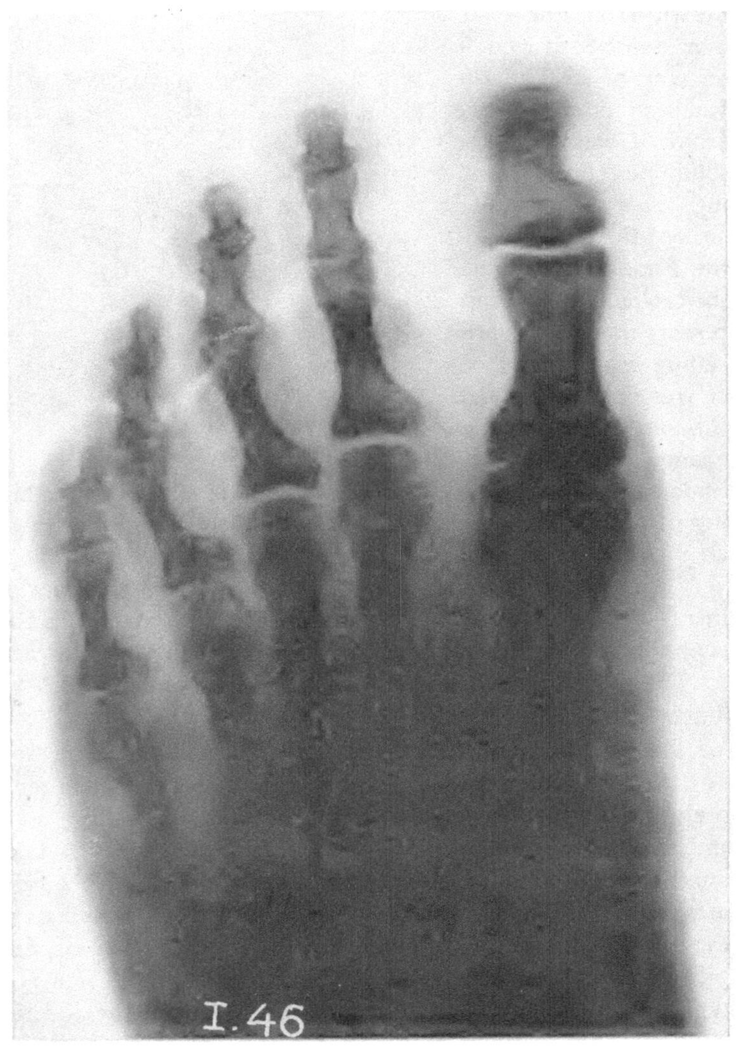

A soldier's foot of exceptionally good type, supporting weight of field equipment, without shoe or sock. (Reduced).

Fig. 32

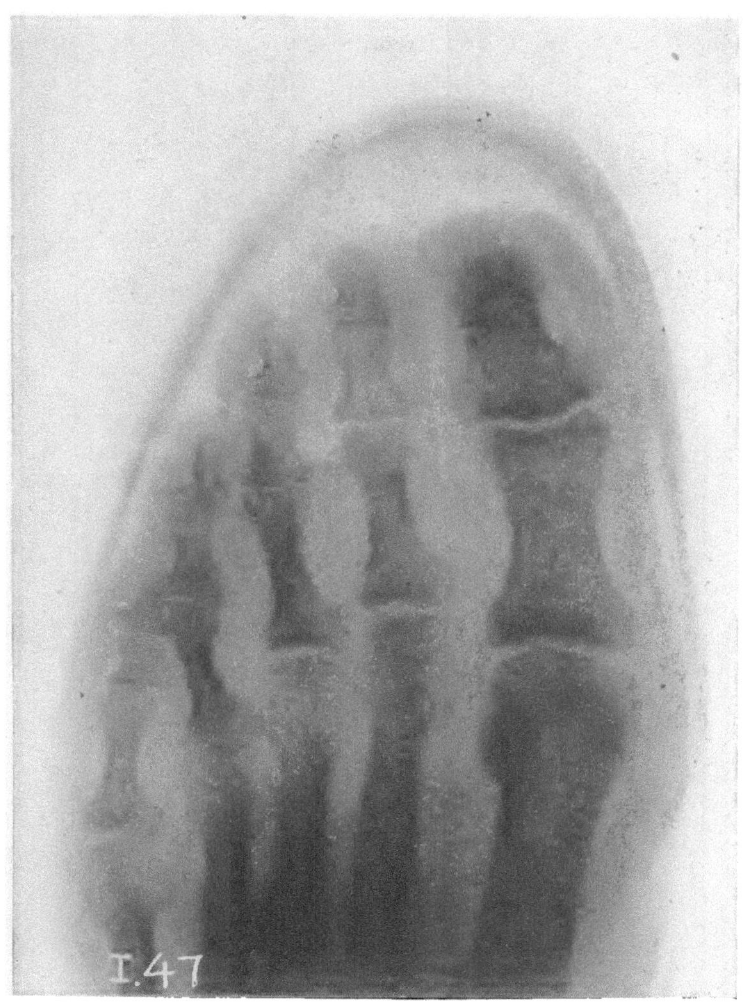

The same foot shown in Fig. 31, supporting weight of full field equipment, but in the garrison tan shoe.

This illustrates a shoe of bad shape, but as good a fit as the shape permits. The soldier was fitted by the Shoe Board. Compare the shape of the foot in this shoe with its own normal, as shown in Fig. 31. (Reduction same as in Fig. 31).

Fig. 33

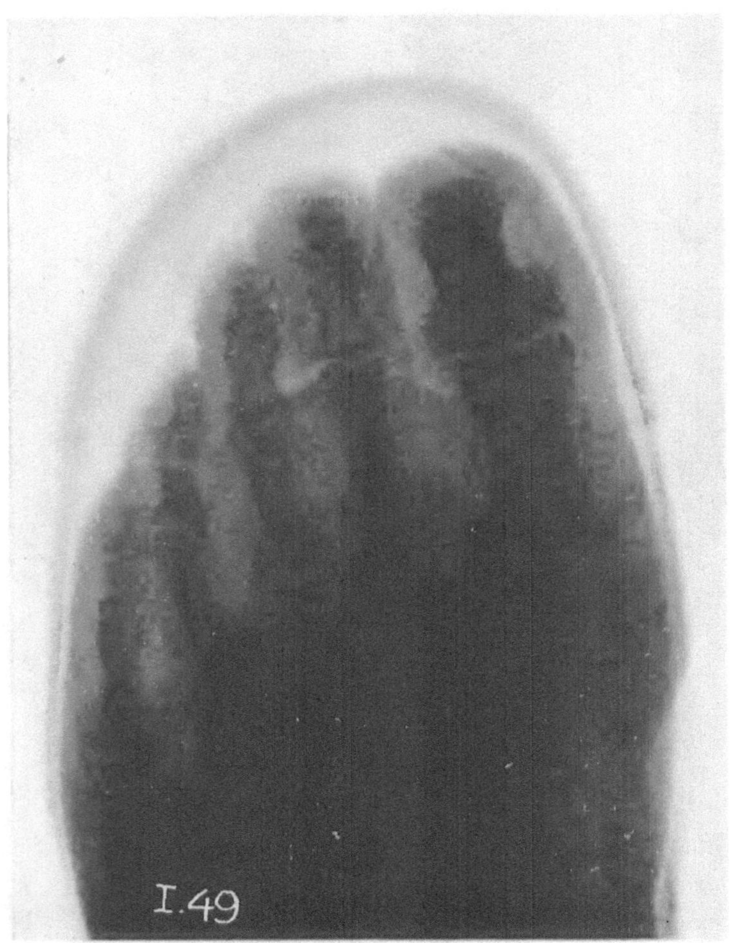

The same foot shown in Figs. 31 and 32, supporting weight of full field equipment but in old style marching shoe.

This illustrates a shoe of bad shape but as good a fit as the shape permits. The soldier was fitted by the Shoe Board.

Fig. 34

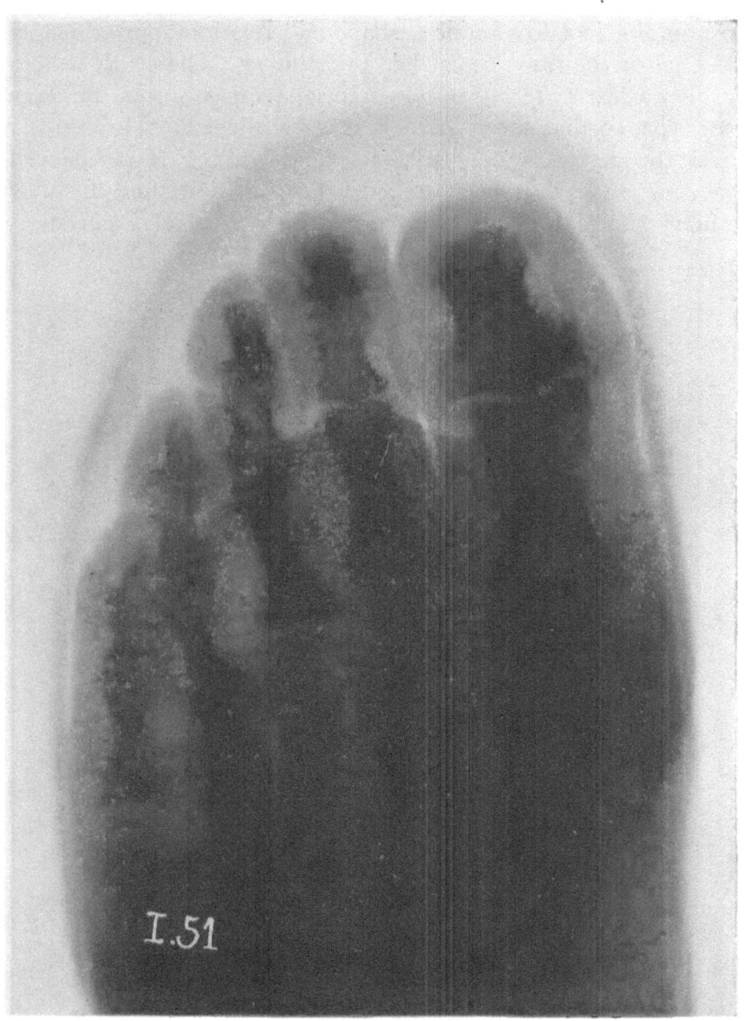

The same foot shown in Figs. 31, 32 and 33, supporting weight of full field equipment, in new military shoe.

This illustrates a good shaped shoe and a perfect fit. **The soldier was fitted by the Shoe Board.**

be seen that the new shoe is the only one of the three which permits the foot to assume a shape and relation approximately like that of the same foot when unconfined. The effort was to develop a last differing in no essential from a normal military foot type, so that shoes built on a certain last would smoothly cover the actual foot of that size and width. It is believed that this effort has been quite successful, and that the new military shoe is the best ever developed for military purposes.

Fig. 35

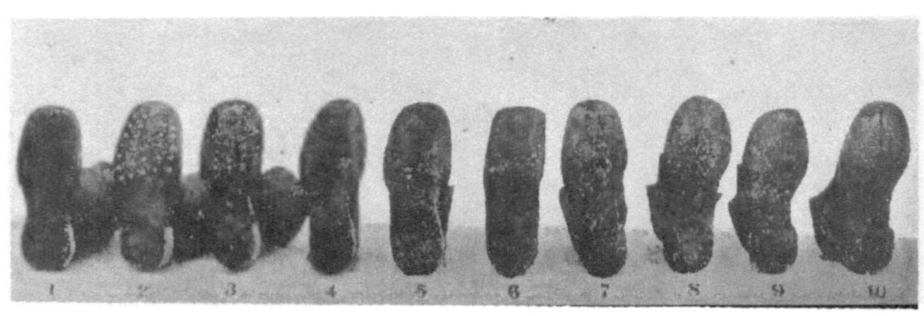

Shape of Sole in various Military Footwear.
(After Melville.)

1. Russian.
2. German (new).
3. German (old).
4. United States, 1908.
5. French.
6. Italian.
7. Japanese.
8. Austrian.
9. Gúrkha.
10. British.

Fig. 36

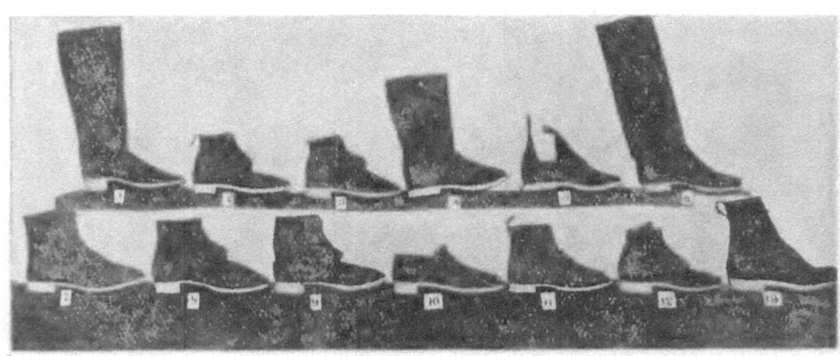

Thickness of Sole and shape of Uppers in various Military Footwear.
(After Melville.)

1. German.
2. British.
3. Gúrkha.
4 and 5. Portugese.
6. Russian.
7. Swedish.
8. Austrian.
9. French.
10. Italian.
11. Japanese.
12. United States, 1908.
13. United States, 1904.

For comparison, attention is invited to Figs. 35 and 36, illustrating the footwear in present use in the armies of all the great military nations. They are evidently very heavy, clumsy and cumbersome as compared with the new United States military shoe. As to shape, their great diversity in this respect indicates that if any one of them is right, all the others must be wrong. As a matter of fact, not a single one of these foreign shoes is physiological in this respect and they may be counted upon to produce unnecessary foot injuries the more they deviate from the anatomical foot type. So bad are they that every military nation, except England and the United States, has to issue a camp shoe to rest the feet of the soldier while in camp. (See Figs. 37 and 38). By issuing a good shoe in the first place, the carriage of this additional burden by the soldier is thus avoided. The Germans, Rus-

Fig. 37

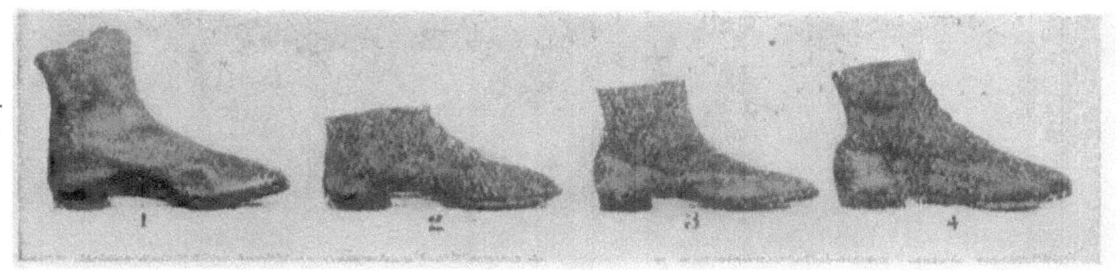

Camp Shoes.
(After Melville.)
1. German (old). 2. German (new). 3. French. 4. Austrian.

Fig. 38

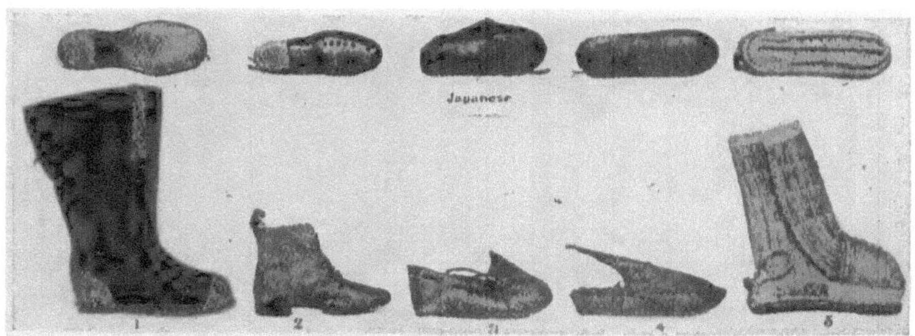

Japanese Foot Gear.
(After Melville.)

sians and Danes still issue high boots, due to the peasantry being used to work in such footwear in mud, wet and snow, with the trousers tucked inside the boot tops.

In concluding this section on the military shoe, it cannot be too strongly emphasized that any deficiencies of shoe supply, or any errors as to fitting, may tend to produce discomfort, dissatisfaction and foot injuries which might erroneously be attributed to the form of the shoe itself. Ideally perfect footwear cannot alone give good results. In other words, the shoe cannot be considered by itself alone, since its actual utility to the wearer depends upon the tripod of supply, fit and construction. If any leg of this tripod fails, the whole structure of foot comfort falls to the ground.

CHAPTER IV.

THE FITTING OF MILITARY SHOES.

A shoe is said to fit when its contour smoothly follows the normal outline of the foot, without undue pressure on any point or points, yet not so loose as to result in harmful friction between the foot and the shoe. These last must thus be considered together, the important thing being the relation between the inner surface of the leather and the outer surface of the skin. The point of support should be large and firm, so as to take up and distribute without injury the shock resulting from the impact of the foot against the ground in marching.

The fitting of the shoes to the feet is the second essential necessary to insuring that the soldier is properly shod. It is of no advantage that a type of shoe be supplied the conformation which very closely approximates the foot type of the soldier, nor would it in addition be of any practical value to have the Quartermaster's Department maintain a full stock of shoe sizes and widths at all posts, unless the shoes selected from the numerous varieties officially available are intelligently chosen and carefully adapted to the requirements of each individual foot. It is a truism to say that when shoes are not properly fitted to feet, those feet will become sore under marching. The fundamental importance of shoe fitting has been largely disregarded in our service, and in every case the fitting of shoes to soldiers should be directly performed by a commissioned officer. The matter of the proper fit of shoes has too close relation to military efficiency to be left to the hazards of chance, indifference, ignorance or prejudice.

There is nothing in the fitting of shoes to the feet of their men which can be regarded as detrimental to the dignity of infantry officers. On the contrary, it is a legitimate part of their duty and direct evidence of their efficiency and desire to enlarge their usefulness. Officers at the Mounted Service Schools learn blacksmithing and farrier's work as part of the regular course; and they learn to themselves fit horse shoes with an intelligent appreciation of the basic influence of proper shoeing upon the marching capacity of cavalry and field artillery. At every post, if a cavalry horse is improperly shod in the production of a bad gait, interference, over-reaching or other fault, the troop commander does not hesitate to give his personal attention to re-shoeing—repeated as often as may be necessary—until the fault has been remedied. Surely the marching capacity of a foot soldier is of quite as much military importance as that of a horse, and the responsibility that it shall be kept at the highest efficiency develops in no less degree upon organization commanders in both instances. Neglect by officers to give proper personal supervision to matters of shoe fitting and supply is equally detrimental to the military efficiency of man and beast.

Criticism of the new military shoe, *per se,* by any person, is thus unjustifiable unless it can first be demonstrated that any injuries to the feet complained of are not the result of improper fitting. It has undoubtedly happened in the past in many cases that footwear has been held responsible by officers and men for foot injuries which were, on the contrary, directly attributable to their own indifference and neglect in the essential matter of fitting.

In fitting the soldier, he should be encouraged to continue to try on shoes until fitted. This, in the past, has not been carried out as properly as should be done. The convenience of those in charge of getting the shoes drawn was apparently more consulted in many instances than the wishes and comfort of the soldier who was to draw them. Any method of fitting which is more or less nominal and perfunctory will be largely barren of the results desired.

In connection with the necessity for properly fitting shoes in the removal of undesirable friction and pressure, it is well to recall the number of completed foot movements required in ordinary marching. Assuming the average step to be 30 inches, each foot will strike the ground at intervals of 60 inches, or every 5 feet. But there are 5,280 feet in a mile, so each foot strikes the ground approximately 1,000 times for each mile traversed. If a fair march for infantry in the field is put at 15 miles, with some 3 miles before and after it in the performance of making and breaking camp and for other purposes, it is evident that each foot will strike the ground some 18,000 times during the day. It is said that falling drops of water will ultimately wear away the hardest stone; and it will be apparent that even a relatively slight defect in the relation between the foot and shoe, if enabled to act with each step through such a vast number of repetitions in such a relatively brief period, can scarcely fail to do injury to the delicate and tender foot structures in contact with it. If the defect be considerable, it is apparent that more or less complete incapacity for marching will scarcely be avoided.

It will probably at once occur to not a few that such careful official supervision by organization commanders of the fitting of the soldier's shoe, as is here laid down, is unnecessary, and that "the soldier is the best judge of what he wants". The latter is undoubtedly true; but it is equally true that in respect to the shoe "the soldier is *not* the best judge of what he ought to wear." And to this statement the officer himself is by no means always an exception. Custom, habit, feet deformed by previous bad shoe selection, desire for conformance with prevailing styles, and regard for conventional ideas of sightliness rather than comfort, so warp the judgment and control the preferences of the average soldier as to make his personal selection of a proper shoe the very rare exception. The Shoe Board, after its careful study of many hundreds of soldiers' feet and its fitting of many thousands of pairs of military shoes, in several of its reports stated its conviction that only about one soldier out of five, if this matter was left to his own selection, would properly fit himself with shoes—and that such proper fits as were actually secured were probably as much the results of chance as of intelligent effort. These conclusions of the board very closely approximated those of Major Reno, M.C., who, in one series of 521 enlisted men of our army studied by him, found that only 26.2% of these wore shoes that were properly fitting; and that in a later series of an additional 609 men, only 16.5% of these men wore shoes that fitted them properly, while 508 had on shoes that did not fit them. In the light of such exhaustive and unbiased studies as have just been mentioned, the propriety from the miltary standpoint of letting the soldier select his own shoes must be emphatically answered in the negative.

In one of its reports the Shoe Board said: "The practical experience of the Board in twice fitting every available man at Fort Sheridan shows absolutely that a very considerable proportion of soldiers cannot be trusted to select their own shoes without guidance and oversight. Some are indifferent, some are slow witted, and many are convinced that a size and width which they believe they have secured before enlistment is the proper size to select in a military shoe. It is the unvarying experience of the board that sizes of shoes suggested by it to such men are accepted by the men as better fitting, after trying on, than were the shoes originally selected by them".

In his lack of judgment in respect to shoe fitting, the soldier is no worse—and is probably better—than the average of men of the military age in civil life. But in his case the effects upon himself of bad selection are so certain, as a result of the necessity for hard marching under heavy burdens not obtaining in civil life, and the aggregate amount of military inefficiency resulting from such cause is so serious, as to demand that a matter of such importance to all concerned shall be taken out of the control of the man himself and reposed in one who, beside having a proper knowledge of what is required, is invested with official responsibility for securing good results. In a general way, it may be stated that the few soldiers found by the Shoe Board to have selected good shoes also had feet exceptionally free from deformity and blemish; this, however, is only what ought to be expected, for if such men had not consistently practiced intelligent selection of shoes, their feet would not have remained good. As the reverse of this rule, it may be accepted that the worse the condition of a

Fig. 39

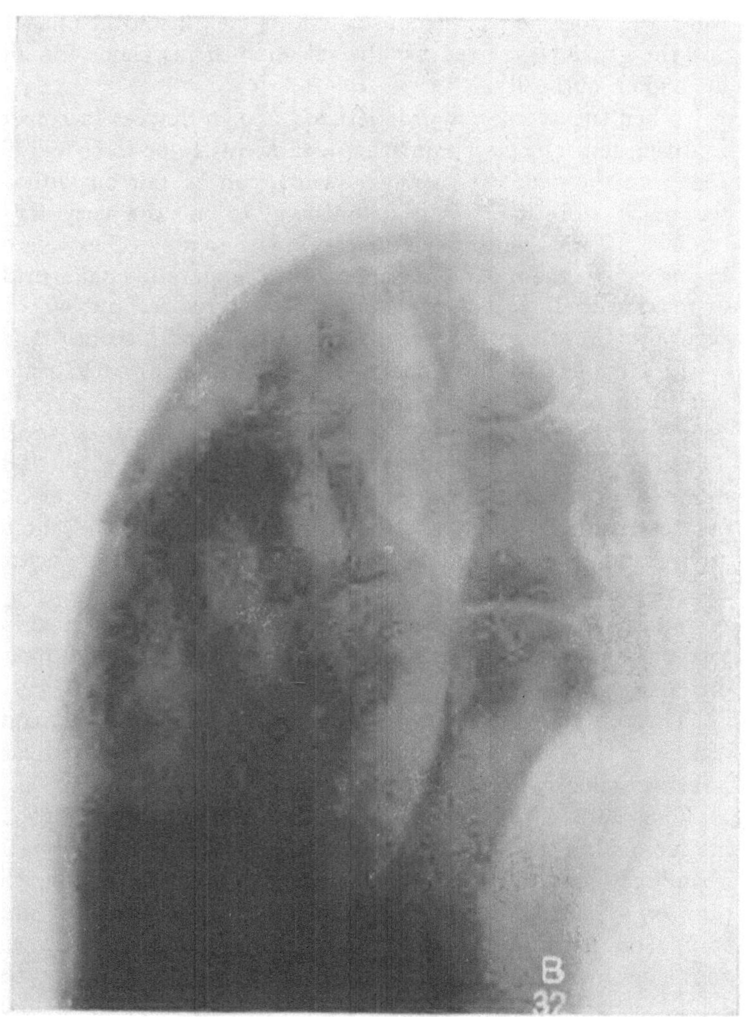

Illustrates defective fitting. Shoe too short and too narrow. Selected by the soldier, whose foot is shown supporting weight of full field equipment.

soldier's feet and the greater the difficulty he has with footwear, the more he has demonstrated his inability to fit himself, and the greater the need for the selection of his shoes for him by higher authority.

When the average man is left to his own devices in respect to fitting himself, his dominating idea seems to be to crowd his foot into the smallest size shoe which can be put on without too much suffering. It is astonishing to see the very large number of men, who, however careless they may otherwise be in respect to their personal appearance, apparently take pride in making their feet appear as small as possible, and who to secure this result will cheerfully accept pain and discomfort.

In the work of the Shoe Board, in one series of 716 men left to themselves in the matter of fitting, 447 or 62½ per cent. found it necessary to try on more than one pair of shoes. The average number of shoes tried on per man was 2.17. The number of trials necessary to secure a fit without previous measurement, but with the members of the board present to advise and suggest, and keep the men trying until an actual fit was secured, was as follows:

1 trial, 269 men; 2 trials, 246 men; 3 trials, 131 men; 4 trials, 35 men; 5 trials, 20 men; 6 trials, 8 men; 7 trials, 4 men; 8 trials, 3 men.

Thus only about a third of a command, under the best conditions of advisory assistance, can be expected to pick out satisfactory shoes without extended trial.

The method the average soldier uses in attempting to fit his feet makes the latter practically impossible to meet the need of military conditions. In this method, the man sits on a bench, puts on the smallest shoe he thinks he can wear, rises and stands on both feet, and takes two or three steps. If his foot does not hurt him too much, the shoe is probably accepted as a fit. His foot has not been permitted to assume even an approximation of its normal degree of expansion and there is no burden on the back to cause the foot to pain under the increased pressure which would be thus created. The soldier thus fits his foot at rest and contracted to its minimum dimensions. He does not know the fact that in marching under the equipment his foot may increase in length and breadth as much as half an inch—and very possibly if he did know he would not care. The result is that a shoe is usually selected which is too tight for light duty in garrison; and in the field compresses the feet, under burden carrying, to an extent which in very many cases may promptly incapacitate for marching. He thus chooses a shoe for considerations of looks under conditions of peace and quiet; the method which the officer must carry out for him has for its purpose the selection of a shoe giving the maximum comfort under conditions of hard field service.

By far the most common fault of shoes which have been selected by the men themselves is insufficient length. Reno found 425 men out of 609 wearing shoes which were too short for them. With shoes of this sort, the toes of the foot, elongating under pressure, are jammed against the front of the shoe in marching, and toe blisters, abrasions and corns are inevitable (See Fig. 39). The next most common fault is insufficient width; of the series of men just mentioned, over twenty-five per cent had mis-fitted themselves in this respect in the probable production of injury in the form of bunions, corns, ingrowing nails, clubbed toes and other defects. (See Fig. 40). Only an insignificant fraction of soldiers, say one or two per cent, tend to select shoes too large for them. These comparative tendencies toward misfit in too small sizes the officers in direct supervision of shoe fitting should bear in mind, so that they may be properly combatted.

Another matter which greatly helps to interfere with securing a fit by the soldier is the fact that shoe lasts have no common standard. Each manufacturer of civilian shoes has his own series of lasts, and all these differ greatly from each other not only in shape but in width. The same applies not only in respect to comparison of civilian and army shoes, but also in respect to the different kinds of army shoes which in the past have been simultaneously supplied. At one time no less than six kinds of shoes, built on totally different lasts, were for issue in our army. All this naturally confuses the soldier lately from civil life. He may recall that the size of a certain brand of civilian shoe which he was accustomed to wear before entering the army, and to which his feet had shaped themselves through long use, was—say—an 8C. He confidently calls for a Government shoe of this size and width, and is surprised on putting it on to find that it in no way feels on his foot like the shoe which he had come to regard as his "size". As a matter of fact, it is totally dissimilar. But, impressed by his previous experience as a civilian, he would very likely draw and attempt to use it. The result in such case will be sore feet, and unsparing and undeserved condemnation of the army shoe as a foot covering.

It is particularly important that young soldiers be given special attention and intelligent guidance in their first shoe fittings after entering the service, so that they may promptly learn the size and width which, in the military shoe, is best adapted to their feet. In this manner also the mistakes as to shoe fitting, found so commonly by the Shoe Board among old soldiers, and so tenaciously adhered to by the latter, would be avoided from the very outset of military life.

Recruits, in time of peace, might be fitted with shoes at recruit depots at the time of their physical examination and the size noted on their descriptive cards. In time of war, old soldiers would draw the sizes and widths of shoes which previous fitting and wear showed to be adapted to their feet. For new organizations and recruits in the field complete sample sets of shoes should be sent to each battalion for fitting.

Another trouble in fitting the shoes in the past has been the requirement that the shoes tentatively selected for trying on by number and letter, had to be taken to barracks for such trying on. It was of course theoretically possible to take back shoes not found to fit and exchange them for another trial size—but distances between barracks and the quartermaster's storehouse were frequently great and the enthusiasm of the soldier to secure what he regarded as a fit notably diminished as several laborious exchanges appeared to be necessary.

Fig. 40

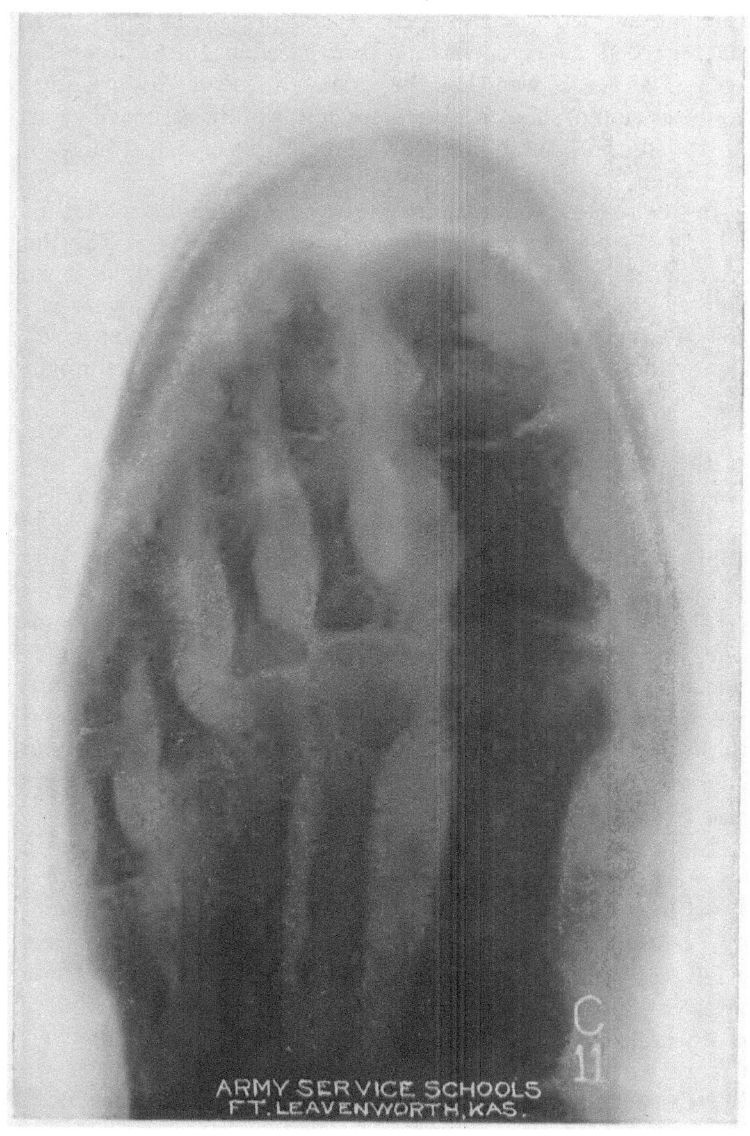

Illustrates defective fitting. Shoe too long and too narrow. Selected by the soldier, whose foot is shown supporting weight of field equipment.

Marching seemed relatively remote and present lack of effort was regarded as compensating for possible future foot injury. The result was that the soldier, in some disgust, ultimately accepted shoes which were not wholly satisfactory to him rather than put himself and others to further trouble in the matter.

In this respect, too, the tendency was to force the soldier into a rapid—even if an unwise—choice, since it was for the convenience of all others concerned in the issue that it be made as quickly as possible. Recruits, particularly, were not infrequently enjoined by superiors to accept what was given them without complaint, even though the shoes so issued might differ widely from what was requested and would fit.

By drawing shoes at the quartermaster's storehouse, under the personal guidance of company officers, the above various causes of administrative defect in shoe fitting are avoided.

The theoretical answer for the question of shoe fitting and supply would be to have the shoes for each man especially built for him upon lasts made from plaster casts of his own feet. This is of course impracticable from the military standpoint, and fortunately it is not at all necessary. Given a shoe as anatomically correct as the one last adopted, always available in fifteen sizes and half sizes with a choice of six different widths for each length, and these fitted with intelligence and judgment, and the problem of foot injuries should largely cease to trouble in our army.

But until a more uniform standard as to feet prevails in the recruiting service, no single pattern of shoe can be expected to exactly meet the needs of all soldiers. A small number of accepted recruits, say one or two per cent, have feet widely variant from the general and normal foot type. These can wear the present shoe, but would very likely be more comfortable in shoes of a somewhat different last. However, if it were attempted to satisfy the needs of this small class in this respect, proportionate discomfort would be produced among a much larger number, for whom the present last is a practical duplicate of their general foot type. Diversity of lasts should not be tolerated in the military service, for the reasons detailed elsewhere. The only reasonable thing to do is to stick to a single last, calculated to afford the greatest good to the greatest number.

The fitting of the soldier with shoes is best done in posts at the quartermaster's storehouse, where proper facilities for trying on should be provided. These include a space of sufficient size, proportional to the strength of the command, so that there need be no unnecessary delay in fitting; benches for the men to sit on while putting on the shoes; a stout box or platform, about two feet high, two feet broad and three feet long, for the soldier to stand upon while being fitted; a quartermaster's foot measure, working in a slotted board so as to give a level surface to the foot being measured; a quartermaster's foot tape measure; one or more quartermaster's shoe stretchers, for the rapid softening and stretching of fitted shoes; a complete set of army shoes, including a sample of every size and width, for fitting by trying on and which orders require that the quartermasters shall maintain at all times; a set of partitioned racks to hold the sample shoes, each space plainly numbered with the size and width of the pair of shoes it is to contain. A copy of General Orders 48, War Department, 1911, or the latest general order, or circular of the Quartermaster General's Office, dealing with the sizes and widths of shoes, and their relation to last measurements, must be available. A chair for the officer to do the fitting, drawn up to the platform on the side which will be on the right of the soldier being fitted, completes the outfit.

All being ready, the soldier to be fitted steps upon the platform in his naked feet, and carrying on his back either the full field equipment with rifle, or a 40 lb. burden to represent approximately the weight of such equipment. This weight is necessary in order to bring about by its pressure the maximum expansion of the soldier's foot, and place it during the shoe fitting under such conditions as it would be placed during marching. While shoe fittings in civil life are habitually based on feet at rest and thus occupying the minimum space in the horizontal plane, the method of shoe fitting here described is based upon the fact that the foot in action differs very materially in appearance and dimension from the foot at rest, and calls for a determination of the greatest length and breadth of the foot under the conditions which regulate its expansion in marching. Conventional ideas as to sightliness control shoe fitting in civil life; those of practical utility and accurate adaptation to each individual normal foot type are intended to govern such fittings in the army. The expansion as to length under conditions of marching pressure is much greater than is ordinarily believed, not a few feet showing a lengthening of as much as one-half of an inch, (compare Figs. 13 and 15) while others grade from that down to a point where lengthening is insignificant. In general, the type of foot showing the greatest expansion as to length is one with a high arch and weak, undeveloped muscles—the least lengthening occurs in strong, normal feet, in which the plantar arch is well filled up with muscular tissue. Flat feet show practically no lengthening whatever, for as the arch is already broken down the foot is incapable of further longitudinal expansion. As the amount of foot lengthening which will result in any individual foot under marching pressure cannot be foretold, it is necessary to produce such expansion, measure the expanded foot, and thereby start the fitting from an accurate individual basis.

In choosing shoes it is necessary first to resort to measurement. Few men know their proper size; others are unwilling, without mathematical demonstration of its necessity, to accept shoes of the dimensions that they ought to wear. Measurement affords assistance to the one and a check on the other. It gives a basic minimum below which shoe sizes, for trying on, should not go. But measurements alone, without trying on, will rarely properly fit a shoe for marching purposes.

To measure the length of the expanded foot, the burdened soldier places his foot on the foot measure working in the slotted board, with the heel in contact with the heel piece of the measure and the great toe lying over the measuring stick. The soldier then stands on his foot, so that the entire weight of the body and the burden being carried is supported by it. He maintains his balance by resting his hand on the shoulder of a comrade, chair-back, or other fixed object. If the latter is not done, attempts to maintain the equilibrium will cause the muscles of the foot and leg to forcibly contract and materially interfere with the relaxation of the foot necessary to its full expansion. The movable block is then pushed in until it just makes contact with the end of the great toe. The measuring stick is graduated in both inches and sizes; for fitting, the former may be disregarded. The size is now read off. Assume, for example, that this size is 6½. If a shoe built on a a 6½ last were put on this foot, the toes would come into direct contact with the front of the shoe, which inevitably would result in toe blisters. To provide sufficient vacant space in front of the toes, two sizes must ordinarily be allowed, making the length of the shoe thus required an 8½. As each size amounts to one-third (⅓) of an inch, the space in front of the toes is thus two-thirds (⅔) of an inch. But putting on the sock reduces this by the thickness of two layers of stocking, one in front of the toes and one behind the heel. Moreover, the foot will slip forward a little in the shoe in marching, especially in going down hill, and when tired and stretched at the end of a march will have elongated to its maximum. Experience has amply demonstrated that an original apparent excess of two sizes is none too much to provide for these contingencies and keep the front of the toes safe from injurious contact with the front of the shoe.

The circumference of the foot around the ball is then taken with the measuring tape. The position of this tape is shown by the line A-B in the accompanying diagram (Fig. 41). The tape is passed snugly around the foot, but not tight enough to compress the flesh and thus spoil the reading. Suppose the tape measure gives a ball measure of 9¼ inches. The length of the shoe required has just been shown to be size 8½. On referring to Circular No. 10, Quartermaster General's Office,

1912, the 8½ column is read down until a ball circumference is found which is the same as that just given by the tape measure. The letter opposite this circumferential measure is then read off. In the present instance, this letter is found to be "D." The size to first try on is thus an 8½ D. But while the length of this shoe is probably correct, its width is still

Fig. 41

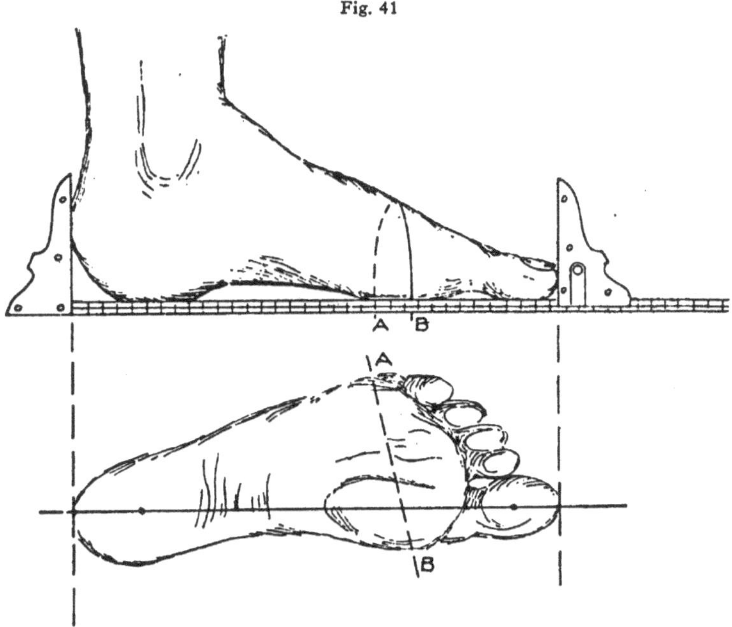

Method of measuring the foot to secure an approximate fit of the shoe to try on.

somewhat problematical and can only be determined by actual, and very possibly repeated, trying on.

It is not necessary, in order to secure a fit, to take the measurements over waist and around heel. These are not essential and may be safely disregarded.

On the number and width of the shoe which these measurements show ought first to be tried being called out, the quartermaster's employee in charge of the fitting room, or other responsible person, takes the pair of shoes in the 8½ D compartment of the sample shoe rack and hands them to the soldier to be fitted. The latter goes to a seat, pulls on a pair of light wool socks, puts on the shoes given him, and laces them tightly. He puts shoes on both feet, for the latter sometimes differ from each other quite materially in size and contour; also sometimes shoes get mixed and the man then receives a mismatched pair. For these reasons, both feet, and not one only, are fitted. The soldier, still with his burden on his back, again mounts the fitting platform. The officer notes with his eye the general appearance of the shoes, as to whether the latter are smoothly adapting themselves to the outline of the feet, are too loose and wrinkling, or are too tight and tense. He then causes the soldier to stand squarely on one foot, supporting himself and his burden or equipment in such a way as to maintain easy equilibrium. The officer then grasps with his hand the vamp of the shoe across its widest part. Bringing his thumb and fingers slowly together, he notes the feel of the leather and its apparent relation to the foot enclosed. If this leather seems loose and tends to wrinkle under the hand, the shoe is too wide and a narrower width should be tried on; if it feels hard, tense and bulging, the shoe is too narrow. A good fit as to width may be said to exist when the foot expanded under body weight has its outline everywhere smoothly followed by the shoe leather, without the latter being either redundant or binding the foot in any manner.

Suitability of length is verified by pressing down the leather in front of the toes. If the leather and tip of the toe touch or are close together the shoe is too short; if more than about a half a thumb's breadth apart, the shoe is too long. In a good fit, there is not less than half an inch of vacant space in front of the great toe under pressure. But clubbed toes, with an elongated second toe protruding beyond the great toe, may in some cases necessitate a greater length in selecting a proper shoe.

Sometimes several trials of different shoes are necessary before a fit is secured, even with careful foot measurement. This is particularly the case with feet presenting some abnormality, as bunions, or hallux with clubbed toes. But the process of trying on must be continued until a fit is secured. Usually it will happen that about twice as many pairs of shoes are tried on as there are men to be fitted.

In connection with this matter of fitting, it is important to remember that each full size differs by one-third ($\frac{1}{3}$) of an inch in length from the next full size; while half sizes, as their name implies, differ from each full size by one-sixth ($\frac{1}{6}$) of an inch. As there are fifteen sizes supplied in our army, there is thus a difference of two and one-half inches in length between the longest and the shortest shoes available. Each letter of width represents one-twelfth ($\frac{1}{12}$) of an inch, and as each size and half size has six widths, a variation of width of half an inch is thus possible for the fitting of each length. With every increase in length by a half size, there is a change in width by one letter—or one-twelfth of an inch. Thus, for example, if a 6D is found to have the right width but to be a little short, a size 6½C should be tried; if a size 8C is of the right width but a full size too long, size 7E would be proper.

It sometimes happens that after a man has been properly fitted as to length, the widest width in that length is found to be somewhat too narrow for him. Under such conditions, a shoe longer than necessary should be given in order to secure the greater width required. A little space in front of the toes does no harm whatever, while a shoe which pinches them will very likely cause discomfort and injury. Mistakes in fitting shoes which are larger than necessary are both rare and little liable to do harm— it is the too short and too narrow shoes which cause the vast majority of injuries and which are to be carefully avoided.

Inasmuch as a flat foot is one in which the maximum elongation has already been practically accomplished, there is relatively little danger of a soldier with such low arch getting a shoe too short for him; but the danger becomes greater and greater according as the soldier's arch is higher and the muscles which support it are thinner and weaker. A high arched but slender and undeveloped foot thus needs an exceptionally long shoe; later, when the foot strengthens, a slightly shorter one may be proper.

The amount of lateral expansion of the foot across the ball, on pressure of body weight and burden carrying, is very considerable. The difference in this respect, between the foot at rest and the same foot under pressure, as demonstrated by radiographs and footprints, amounts in many feet to as much as half an inch. (See Figs. 13 and 15). Feet which have been squeezed and contracted by too narrow shoes usually show a relatively greater proportion of foot expansion in weight carrying than feet already well expanded through use of good footwear. (See Figs. 42 and 43). This stretching naturally tires and renders painful the transversalis and interosseous muscles through their entire extent. Such stretching and discomfort does not mean that the shoe is wrong, but it does mean that the foot itself is at fault as a result of improper footwear previously worn. And it is a very cogent argument for the use of but one last—and that a physiological one—by the soldier.

Another reason for fitting the shoe large, besides its natural expansion, is the fact that the foot swells considerably in prolonged marching, through flow of blood to the part and interference with its return flow from pressure on the veins. Then the constant striking of the foot against the ground is a stimulus to the flow of blood to that part, with dilation of the capillaries, just as a red mark follows a blow on the flesh of any other part of the body. After hard marching, the soles of the feet are often painful and reddened from this cause; and with shoes which are too small, the soldier in marching in warm weather has a feeling of heat and irritation in his feet from congestion due to such interference with the circulation; in the winter, on the contrary, the same cause operates to make the feet cold, numb and readily susceptible to frost bite.

The number of shoe sizes and widths now officially provided is undoubtedly quite sufficient to meet the needs of all soldiers' feet except the very few enlisted with feet widely variant from the generally military foot type. Thus in one ser-

Fig. 42

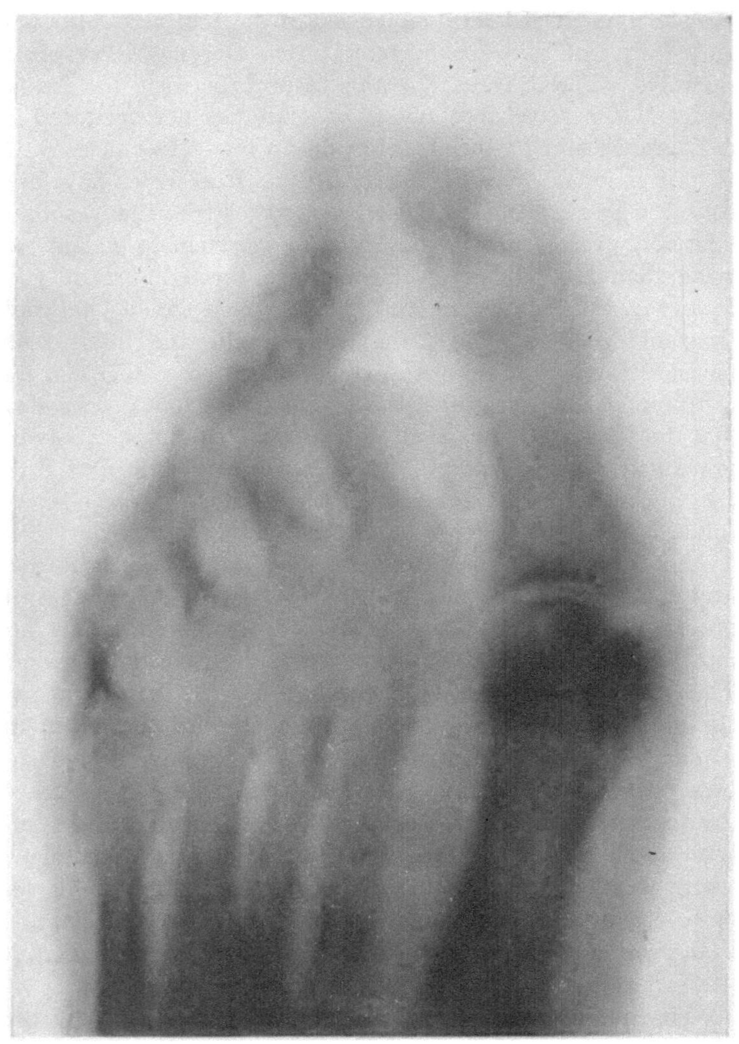

Soldier's foot badly deformed by too tight shoes. Foot is at rest as the soldier is seated.

Fig. 43

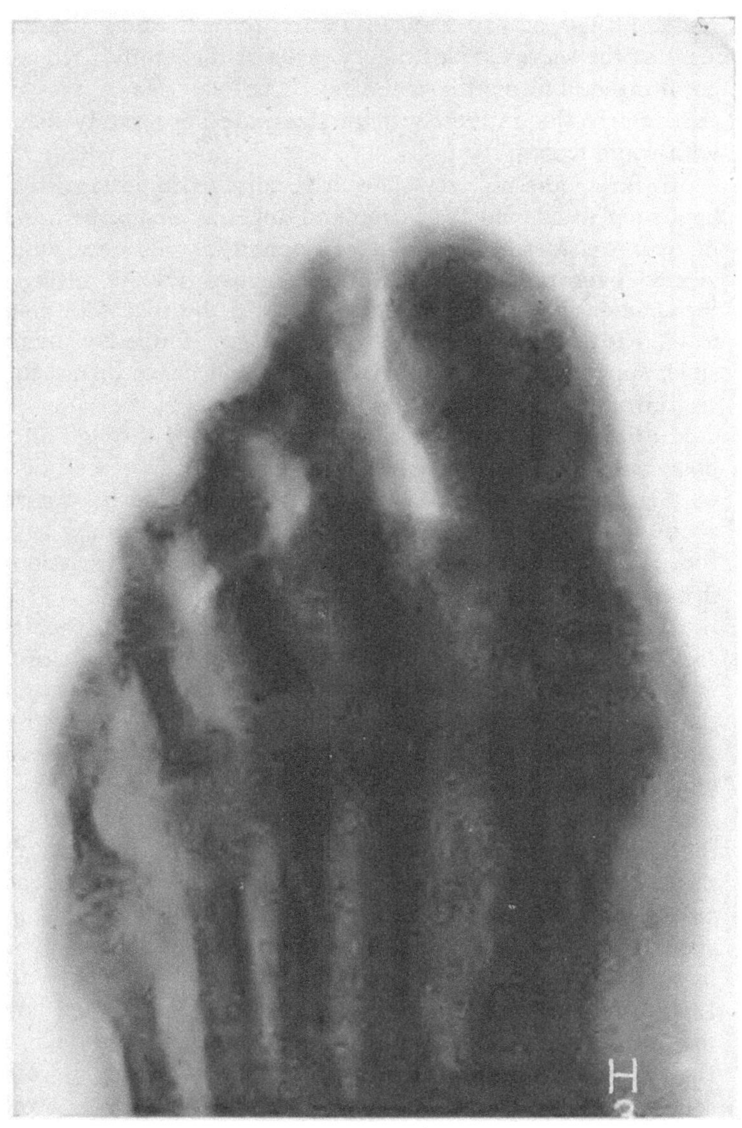

Same foot shown in Fig. 42, but the soldier is now supporting his weight on this foot.

ies of fittings of 716 men, in a garrison containing the three arms of the service, 23 of the 75 varieties then authorized were not utilized in fitting the command. The extremes of sizes, and particularly the extremely large sizes, are very rarely needed with white troops.

In fitting the military shoe, it is quite as important that it be a snug fit around the instep and ankle as that it be a loose fit over the toes. The point of support in this new shoe is located over the instep, and this requires smooth fitting of the shoe over the posterior three-fifths of the foot with ability to hold it firmly in position by its lacing. If this be not possible, slipping of the shoe on the foot will occur in marching and injury to the latter is certain.

In fitting the shoe, the laces must be passed through all the holes and tied after being well tightened. A shoe well fitting in this respect will usually have the margin of its quarters about one-half inch apart when well laced. According as the foot is greater or less developed than the average, variation in this marginal interspace will naturally occur.

It is important that the position of the shoe on the foot, as a whole, be stable. This is best accomplished by a close fit in the posterior half of the foot, in which lateral pressure on the sides of the heel, and around the heel over the front of the ankle joint, can cause no interference with any structure intended to be mobile.

In a small percentage of soldiers, the proper fitting of the military shoe is rendered quite difficult by the fact that they have relatively large, broad feet, low insteps and slender ankles. For this class, which is fortunately small in number, a shoe that is large enough for the lower part of the foot is too large to properly fit the upper foot and ankle. The latter fault is serious, since unless the foot can be held snugly over the instep and ankle against slipping about in the shoe on the march, foot injury is practically certain. In a few other soldiers, a shoe at first apparently satisfactory may so stretch in the uppers as to be no longer capable of lacing snugly. A practical way of remedying these defects is to insert one or more thicknesses of blanket, cloth, or felt, torn into suitable strips, between the tongue and lacing of the shoe, so that the latter, when pulled tight, may thus have a point of firm support by which it can keep the foot in its proper position in the shoe. Occasionally, with an extremely slender, low instep, it may be well to pull the laces snugly and tie them in a knot at the third or fourth eyelet; this supports the shoe better, and looseness in the last two or three holes is of less importance as regards foot injury.

The average soldier may be expected to object more or less vigorously to the size and width of the shoe given him under his first fittings by his company commander. Accustomed as he has been to shoes which constantly bind and compress his feet, he will regard the new shoe given him as too long and too loose. The squeezing of his feet by the shoes he has himself habitually chosen has been so long continued as to appear to him to be natural and necessary. Hence any complaints that the shoes are unduly large should be looked upon with doubt, and should be disregarded unless corroborated by the officer in charge by the actual manipulation of the shoe and foot by the method already described. In the fittings made by the Shoe Board, a large number of protests of this nature were made at the time that the shoes were issued and during the first day or so of the march test. It was noted that these complaints practically disappeared by the time the march test was half over; and in no single instance during the foot examinations, when the man complained of his shoes being too large, did his feet show any evidence of injury whatever. It is nearly always too small shoes, and not what may feel at first like too large ones, that cause sore feet. Beside fitting shoes to his men, the officer is thus called upon to combat error, prejudice and misconception. The relations between foot and shoe, which constitute a proper fit, are excellently shown in Fig. 34.

Where there is any difficulty in accomplishing a fit, it must be borne in mind that the trouble may not necessarily be in the shoe but may be in the foot itself, through some abnormality causing it to vary from the general type.

In these trials of shoes, any local conditions affecting their fitting will be noted. Hurtful local pressure over bunions and corns can usually be seen and always can be determined by the hand. The same applies to pressure over the great toe. The man himself should be questioned, and any area or point of the shoe which is said to cause discomfort should be carefully examined. Sometimes such a shoe is badly finished, is shrunken from having been taken off the last too soon, or has a rough seam or wrinkled lining inside.

It must be remembered that the shoe is built over a last which has perfectly smooth surfaces and gently curving contours such as are not found in the human foot. The last, while perhaps quite accurately reproducing in the transverse plane the sectional area of the foot at any given point, thus only relates to sectional bulk and general outline. The latter, in a generally fitting shoe, may both be quite correct, and yet the shoe may cause discomfort and foot injury. The reason is that it as yet is only partially fitted and still requires to be adapted to local conformation of the foot. If the latter presents no material abnormalities, this adaptation can be gradually accomplished by occasional and progressively lengthened periods of wear, until the shoe is "broken in"—in other words, until the stretching over the prominences of the foot resulting from use of the shoe has resulted in better equalization of pressure, with enlargement where needed at the expense of contraction where excess of leather is unnecessary. But it must be emphasized that the process of "breaking in" is not without some risk that the foot, and not the shoe, will "break in" first. The foot injuries so commonly seen in soldiers have almost invariably had their beginning in just such attempts to "break in" new shoes, which, in either size, shape or both, did not approximate the foot expected to wear them.

Very much of the danger of such foot injury can be avoided by the use, on shoes found proper as to length and width but which are still not wholly comfortable to the feet of the wearer, in the fitting room or barracks, of the shoe stretchers provided by the Quartermaster's Department.

This type of shoe stretcher is practically a last made in two longitudinal halves, capable of being forced apart to the extent desired after being inserted in the shoe. This type is particularly adapted to stretching the leather across the toes as a whole, and is capable of giving the shoe upper a shape quite different from what it had acquired when taken off the last. This stretcher is provided with holes in both its last halves, so located as to come approximately in the foot areas especially liable to pressure, blisters, corns and bunions. Adjustable bulbs, with pegs to go in these holes and hold them in proper position, are provided to accomplish local stretching and relief from pressure. After marking with a pencil on the outside of the shoe the points of painful pressure, one or more bulbs are put in position under them and the leather forcibly stretched. For very large or sensitive bunions and corns, the use of this stretcher is quite satisfactory, for the areas to be treated can be thoroughly wetted to facilitate stretching of the leather and the apparatus left in the shoe over night. A very free use of this stretcher in the shoes just selected is nearly always advisable and does nothing but good.

It sometimes happens that shoes, after partial stretching, tend to return to their original form and become uncomfortable. To avoid or remedy this, the subsequent periodical use of the shoe stretchers, which are authorized for issue to each company, should be enjoined on their men by organization commanders in all cases where relief from shoe pressure is required.

A very excellent method of adapting the shoes to the feet, after careful fitting of the latter, consists in having the man stand in his shoes in about three inches of water for about five minutes, or until the leather becomes thoroughly wet and pliable and in condition to stretch easily. The soldier then walks on a level surface for about an hour, or until the shoes have dried on his feet, to the shape of which the pressure of body weight and muscular action have forced the leather in drying to conform. If desired, a little neatsfoot oil may be rubbed on the shoes to keep them supple after taking them off, but this procedure is not necessary. Shoes treated in this way are made as comfortable in an hour—and without any possible danger of injury to the feet—as could be done with a week's wear under the ordinary method of "breaking in". This method is particularly necessary and valuable where troops are issued new shoes which there is no time to break in slowly before they must be used for marching. It can be properly used under any conditions except when the temperature is well below freezing; and even then can often be carried out to a less complete but still advantageous extent by wearing the damp shoes indoors. The method does the shoe no harm, and merely secures with intent the beneficial results which would happen in any case through the first rain in which the shoes are worn. It is a deliberate repetition of the method originally employed to make the leather adapt itself to the last in shoe manufacture, and which is again employed to make the leather of the resulting shoe conform to the local contours of the foot which it must subsequently enclose and protect.

If the soldier has drawn and stretched shoes which, from some foot malformation, are still uncomfortable, a new effort for fitting must be made. In all probability the company records will show other men fitted by the same size and width who will be able to take over and use the offending shoes. But it is far better to throw away shoes which do not fit than to keep them at the expense of probable serious foot injury. If the foot deformity is of such a nature as to prevent fitting, it disqualifies the soldier for further military service.

The recruit will probably need two especially careful shoe fittings, one as soon as he enters the service and a second one some six months later. It is a matter of observation of the Shoe Board that the foot of a recruit put in the army shoe tends to broaden, thicken and strengthen very materially after enlistment through use of a broader last and the foot development resulting from marching and other exercise. A shoe somewhat different in width from that originally selected will very likely now be found to be desirable. But after the feet are once expanded and "set", further change of shoe will not be necessary and the man's shoe size becomes practically a constant quantity for future requisitions and trials.

After the military shoe has been fitted to the newly enlisted recruit, the latter should not undertake hard marching in it for at least a fortnight. This requirement, for a shoe which is properly fitted, may seem strange. But the army shoe is built on a last quite different from that of the shoe which the recruit has worn until recently and to the shape of which his foot has become habituated and conformed by long use. The army last is broader, its shape is dissimilar and its points of support are different from the ordinary civilian shoe. The result is that the foot of the recruit must be given time to adapt itself to its new covering. Its outline must be altered, new bearing surfaces must be toughened, and—most important of all—foot muscles hitherto weak and undeveloped must be strengthened to support ligaments now subjected to a greater and unaccustomed strain. It takes time, of course variable with the individual, to do all this; but until such alteration and improvement of the foot type has been accomplished, discomfort and dissatisfaction with the new shoe may be expected on hard marching.

In the second fitting of the recruit with shoes, and in old soldiers, no such objections exist in respect to the immediate use of new shoes in the field, for the foot has by this time been changed in the above respects.

The practice, heretofore very common, of wearing the garrison or a civilian shoe about the post, and then abruptly putting on a marching shoe built on a totally different last for marching at occasional intervals, is most inadvisable. Under such methods, the foot is periodically forced to attempt a temporary variation in type, with resulting discomfort and foot injury. (See Figs. 32, 33 and 34). The supply by the Government of several different kinds of shoes is thus most undesirable, and permission to wear civilian shoes while in uniform should be withheld by company commanders. All shoes worn by soldiers should be made on one last—and one last only. For garrison and field work the shoe should be the same. It is undoubtedly much better to stick to a single last, even if the latter were somewhat imperfect, than to alternate the use of a shoe built on excellent lines with another built on a last of dissimilar character.

CHAPTER V.

SHOE SUPPLY.

It should be almost superfluous to say that after determining the proper size and width of shoe required to fit the individual soldier, no shoe other than that thus determined to fit should be accepted for him except in great emergency. In garrison, it will usually be possible to delay drawing until a fitting size can be obtained. In case of necessity, a shoe too large rather than one too small should be selected; for a shoe too large in its several dimensions may be made quite comfortable by the use of heavy woolen socks or several pairs of light ones. However, the soldier himself, if given a preference under such conditions, will usually choose the small one. The frequently considerable shortage of stock of shoes kept on hand at posts has, in the past, resulted in very many instances of unnecessary foot injury through the soldier having to draw a shoe which did not fit, or go without any. Ill fitting shoes forced upon the soldier in this way are certain to do him harm. There is, of course, no necessity for such requirement, for shortage of stock in this fundamentally important respect can and should be anticipated and prevented by every efficient quartermaster. General Orders 26, War Department, 1912, require that special written report shall be made by organization commanders to their post commanders in each case where the sizes and widths of shoes requisitioned for are not available or the official facilities for fitting them are not provided; post and other commanders are to investigate and take such appropriate remedial action on these reports, as lies in their power; also the latter are to furnish a record of the number of such reports, and the reasons for such deficiencies, to inspectors at each inspection of the post.

Inspections conducted under the provisions of Paragraph 913, Army Regulations, are to embrace an inquiry into the manner in which the foregoing order has been complied with, and the report of inspections is to include a statement of all instances of failure on the part of company commanders to secure proper shoes for their commands, and the cause of such failure. This should do much to cause proper forethought in maintaining at all times a sufficient shoe supply.

It is also required that post quartermasters shall maintain a full series of shoes, including a sample of every size and width, for use by organizations in fitting by trying on. This series is to be kept intact and suitable for trying on by returning to the general stock for issue any shoes beginning to stretch from use and alter in appearance from handling. By the use of this series of samples, shoes may be fitted and appropriate requisition thereby made for such varieties as may be needed and are not on hand.

This matter of completeness of stock from which to make fittings and draw shoes is a matter of fundamental importance. No matter how carefully efforts to fit the man's feet are made, it is obvious that unless the special variety of shoes needed by him are on hand for supply, the soldier can not be provided with suitable footwear. Shortage of shoe supply is a matter of administrative incapacity which cannot be tolerated by company commanders, as having too direct and profound an influence on the military efficiency of their organizations.

If a civilian desires a certain size and width of shoe he can go to a second shoe store if he cannot obtain what he desires in the first one. The soldier, however, has no second source of supply to which he can, or would be allowed to, resort. He must take what is given him. If the local quartermaster's supply is deficient, the soldier must do without what he wishes and requires and what the Government is supposed to supply to him.

In connection with the matter of supply, the Shoe Board, in 1912, called for data from five large posts, including the largest in the army, in respect to the number, length and width of all the marching shoes supposed to be kept in stock and available for issue. Of these, one post lacked 9 per cent; another

18 per cent; another, 27 per cent; another, 47 per cent; another, 85 per cent. Not only was there such shortage as would render fitting of soldiers impossible, but as it was chiefly in the sizes in most common use which were most frequently drawn, those which remained were largely off sizes capable of fitting but a small proportion of the command.

It is quite conceivable that about any article other than shoes could be ill fitting and still be worn by the soldier without particular discomfort or detriment to his military efficiency. An ill fitting pair of trousers or shirt would have no particular influence on the performance of field duty, though appearances might suffer somewhat. But in respect to shoes, he must have exactly the length and width of shoes his feet require, or pay an undeserved penalty which is exacted not only from the man himself but falls in large part upon the Government which employs him.

It may be true that the supply department has certain administrative restrictions which interfere with the maintenance at all times of a full assortment of shoes in posts. But the same authority which created these artificial restrictions is competent to remove them. Economy in the military service is of course desirable, but the last item on which to make a saving is the soldier's shoe. Every post should have its surplus stock of shoes sufficient to meet the needs of any reasonable anticipation. Recruits are liable to arrive at any time—or troops, whose proper requisitions have been sent in at one station, are suddenly sent to another before supply. Experience will in time furnish accurate information as to the number of pairs of shoes of each size and width required in the fitting of United States soldiers, and proper use of such information in advance should ordinarily forestall any shortage of stock. Much data of this sort has been tabulated in the past by the Quartermaster's Department, but as this relates to shoes built on lasts now obsolete and quite different from those now used, and to shoe issues based on unsupervised choice by soldiers and not on their careful fitting, such data is practically valueless for present purposes. It will not take long, however, to secure for supply purposes sufficient new data based on modern shoes and readjusted conditions.

According to figures given by Reno in respect to the sizes of shoes worn by 521 men examined by him, only about one pair of shoes in sizes, 5, 5½, 6, 9½, 10, 10½, 11 and 11½ are required for every seven or eight pairs required in the medium

Fig. 44

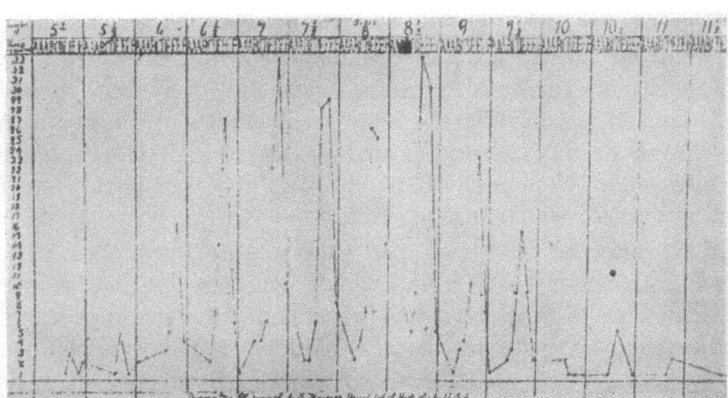

Chart illustrating the proportion of shoe sizes ordinarily drawn. (From Reno.)

sizes of 6½, 7, 7½, 8, 8½ and 9. His figures, expressed in graphic form, appear in Fig. 44.

Shoe supply must also take cognizance of other modifying factors in respect to the proportion of each variety of shoe to be kept in stock. These have to do with race, for colored troops habitually require shoes averaging a size or more larger than white troops of the same branch of the service. The Filipino troops, conversely, being small men, will find their shoe fittings in the small sizes. The composition of a force or garrison, by branch of service, must also be given consideration; for cavalrymen, for example, are smaller men, have smaller feet, and can wear a more snug fit than the infantry by reason of using their feet less and carrying less burden; while artillery men of the mountain batteries, in whom a minimum height of 68 inches is required, have feet proportioned in size to the greater size of these men. All these facts can and should be considered by quartermasters in submitting their estimates for shoe supply, and sincere co-operation with company commanders in assuring that every man of the command is properly shod should be the rule.

But it may be that some contingency has resulted in shortage of certain varieties of shoes desired. There must be some way of getting these shoes without delay, for the soldier needs his shoes at once. As quartermasters are officially responsible for so many pairs of shoes merely, without regard to length and width, it should be quite possible for them to have authority to mail back to depot quartermasters a sufficient number of surplus sizes and receive by return mail the same number of shoes of the missing sizes required. This arrangement would produce no undesirable complications as to property responsibility, would tremendously facilitate prompt and proper shoe supply, and would enable stock provided on the basis of a different size and composition of the command to be properly adjusted to present needs by turning in shoes from sizes which, under changed conditions, may have become largely superfluous.

But whatever administrative obstacles may arise to interfere with efficient shoe supply, they must be removed. No matter of departmental method or convenience must be permitted to remain which in any way can interfere with such a matter of fundamental military importance as the shoeing of the soldier.

CHAPTER VI.

THE CARE OF THE FEET.

Field Service Regulations, paragraph 142, prescribe that in the management of marching troops "special care is paid to the feet". While details of the necessary "care" cannot of course be given in a work of that general nature, it is believed that the care of the soldier's foot, like his selection of a shoe, has been given far less official regard than its importance deserves; under the specious reasoning that if the soldier did not look out for the welfare of his own feet he would find appropriate punishment in the results of his own neglect. This idea is of course faulty in that it apparently overlooks the fact that the soldier is not always informed as to the best procedure for the care of his feet, and that some need oversight and direction to spur them on to proper effort; it also ignores the fundamental fact that the interest of the Government, which demands that nothing shall be left undone which can make the soldier more efficient as a fighting unit, is paramount. Better appreciation of this necessity is the basis of the greater official care given the feet of the soldier in foreign armies. It is probably also generally true that the regulation requiring personal inspections of the men is interpreted by the majority as being primarily directed at the detection of certain contagious diseases, and that the coincident foot inspection is relatively superficial and perfunctory. This attitude is unfortunate, for so long as infantry is the backbone of an army and mobility is the most important element in strategy, frequent careful inquiry into the condition of the feet, and constant interested oversight looking to their continued welfare, are properly to be required of all officers concerned. This duty is not always congenial, but the same is true of various other necessary things connected with the military service.

And probably no one thing will more conduce to greater marching radius, the success of tactics, and the delivery on the firing line of the maximum number of rifles, than will proper foot care of the command. Conversely, neglect in this respect produces a vast amount of military inefficiency.

The remedying among their men of minor defects, like their prevention, largely falls within the province of organization commanders as being part of the legitimate internal administration of the company. For this duty, no more technical knowledge is required than may properly be expected of all officers with foot troops. Only in relatively few cases should the professional advice and assistance of the surgeon be required, when the company officer possesses and applies a reasonable and proper knowledge as to foot conditions and foot care. The view that minor defects should habitually be treated by the surgeon is quite incorrect.

The officer in command of foot troops is just as directly concerned in the maintenance of good condition of the feet of his men as is the cavalry officer in the good condition of the feet of his horses. The latter causes the hoofs of his animals to be cleaned out and inspected twice daily, frequently looks into their condition himself, and sees that any faulty shoeing, causing interference, over-reaching or stumbling is promptly rectified. No such constant attention to the feet of his men would be required of the infantry officer, but this is no reason why practically no attention at all should be given by him to this matter. Only a couple of shoe fittings and periodical foot inspections are necessary for him in order to keep his command in good marching condition. It is quite as essential to military efficiency that men shall be as well shod as are horses, and that corns and other minor foot defects in the former shall be as well prevented and intelligently treated, under the direction of company commanders, as in the latter. Nor is the habitual advice and assistance of the surgeon and veterinarian necessary in either case.

If the company commander gives due care to the careful fitting to shoes of newly arrived recruits, and repeats this in a few months when their feet have altered in shape and developed in size and strength, as a result of the use of the physiological army shoe and practice in marching under burden carrying, he will probably subsequently need to give his men little further attention in this respect other than to see that they fit on and draw the size and width with which they were last fitted, and counteract the general tendency to secure a shoe too small for the needs of the foot in marching.

But he must verify, by frequent foot inspections, the fact that the shoes thus selected really do fit, and at the same time he should give such simple, common sense directions as should result in the relief or removal of the ordinary foot defects. For the making of these foot inspections, as with the routine examination of animals on the picket line, the presence of the surgeon and veterinarian, as already mentioned, is unnecessary. Only in a very few instances will medical advice and assistance be required, and these doubtful cases should be sent to the surgeon for examination.

The necessary frequency of foot inspections is variable with conditions. In barracks, when men are marching but little, one such inspection every fortnight should meet all needs. But in the field, or when troops are undergoing hard marching, such inspections should be made daily, that trifling defects and injuries may be given prompt attention and thereby prevented from developing into matters of importance.

The time required to make the foot inspection of a company is not to exceed half an hour, and as officers and men become accustomed to the routine it may be shortened to half that time. For two officers of a company working independently, such an inspection is a matter of only a very few minutes. Never under any circumstances does it approach in duration the time required for the "stables" held twice a day by a mounted command.

The inspection is made after the feet have been washed; in many cases it is combined with the general inspection of the person required by regulations. In garrison, the men stand in bare feet at the foot of their bunks until the officer has passed them by; in the field, they sit on the ground in front of their tents, or at such other convenient place as may be required. As the officer passes, accompanied by the non-commissioned officer in charge, he notes the condition of the feet, especially in regard to recent injury but also with reference to old remediable defects. In case that attention to the feet is needed, he gives appropriate directions to the soldier in the presence of the non-commissioned officer, who becomes responsible for their being carried out.

Fig. 45

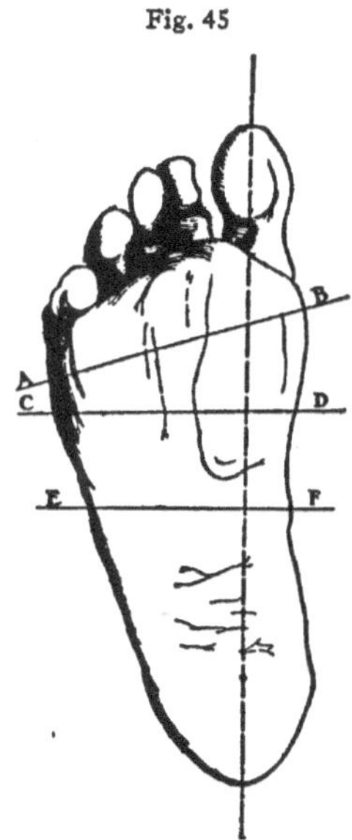

A well shaped foot. The vertical line is "Meyer's line" and is the measurement for foot length; A-B is the ball measure; C-D is the waist measure; E-F is the high instep measure.

The general condition of the feet of foot troops who have not received proper attention may be stated to be bad. In his analysis of the feet of 609 men, Reno found 64 men, or about 10 per cent, the condition of whose feet he was willing to class as good. In this he was either more fortunate or liberal than the Shoe Board, who did not regard as being of good character the feet of half that percentage in the many men it examined. He classified some abnormalities found in this series, which when summarized, gave the following results:

Callosities, cases (number in multiple callosities not given)	81
Callosities; jamming of toes	121
Callosities; ingrowing nails	19
Callosities; jamming of toes; hammer toes	31
Jamming of toes	29
Jamming of toes; ingrowing nails	94
Ingrowing nails	23
Callosities; jamming of toes; bunions	23
Callosities; bunions	10
Callosities; deformed nails	3

Callosities; jamming of toes; ingrowing nails	78
Flat feet	2
Total cases of serious foot blemish	514

Beside the above conditions, the foot deformity known as hallux valgus was so common as practically to be universal and to a degree materially influencing marching capacity. Compare Figs. 45 and 46.

Fig. 46

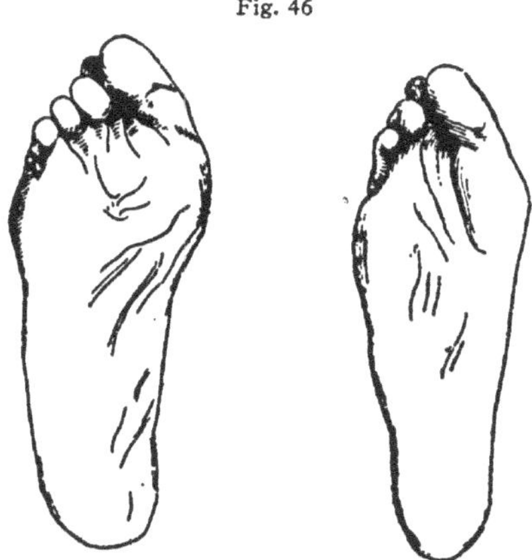

Deformities of Feet Resulting from Bad Shoes.

The experience of the Shoe Board closely tallies with the tabulation by Reno, that more than ninety out of every hundred enlisted men had foot defects which more or less interfered with marching and needed attention and rectification.

There is no question but that the company commander who is fully appreciative of his duties and responsibilities will be astounded and somewhat dismayed at the results of a careful and critical foot inspection of his men.

With respect to the vast amount of foot blemish now present in our army, all but a very small proportion of it is removable by the simple measure of selecting a shoe which closely resembles the normal contour of the average foot, and fitting it on the latter with due regard for proper length and width. With relief from harmful pressure, corns and callouses, primarily developed—but now no longer needed—as protective agencies, will be largely cast off; ingrown nails tend to straighten and cease to pain; hallux valgus and bunions begin to correct themselves. A few simple additional agencies, as later detailed, materially assist in this improvement. Such few severe blemishes as do not yield are subjects for the attention of the surgeon or discharge on surgeon's certificate of disability.

Beside official oversight, the men themselves must be required to give attention to their individual foot care. They must be required to report foot injury without delay, and those who fail to do this should be made to march. In very many instances, it will be found that the infantry soldier who lets his feet get sore is quite as much to blame as the mounted soldier who lets his horse's back get galled.

For their better recognition by officers and non-commissioned officers of the line, a brief description of the several foot defects commonly found in soldiers, with simple measures for their improvement and cure, here follows.

Hallux Valgus.

This name is given to the common condition in which the great toe is pushed away from its proper straight inner line and made to join in its several bones, and these with its metatarsal bone, at a more or less considerable angle. It is well shown in Figs. 42, 46 and 47. It is produced by shoes which have an outward bend and not a straight inner line to the last. If the improper curve of the inner margin of the sole begins well back, the hallux valgus commences at the metatarso-phalangeal joint and if the deviation is considerable a bunion will probably result. If the outward curvature of the last begins well toward the front, it is the further bone in the toe which is bent away, while the second bone remains in nearly its proper alignment; this pressure on the side of the tip of the toe being especially the cause of ingrowing nail. Since nearly all civilian shoes of a fashionable type have a crooked last, it follows that hallux valgus, of greater or less degree, is present in the vast majority of soldiers. In fact, it is so common and well established among them that the board which devised the recent army shoe was compelled to take a certain degree of it into consideration as being a "normal abnormality".

The degree of interference with marching capacity which hallux valgus produces, depends upon the angle of deviation which the everted toe makes with its proper axis. The latter is represented by the socalled "Meyer's Line", which in the normal, undeformed foot starts from the tip of the great toe and passes as a straight line through—and parallel with—the long axis of the great toe and, continuing on, emerges from the heel at its central point. Such a normal foot and line is shown in Fig. 45. This straight line, running from toe to heel, indicates a vertical plane through which is secured the strongest mechanical support to the body weight, the most effective thrust of the foot, and the greatest anatomical efficiency of the attached muscles.

In some cases of hallux valgus, the great toe may deviate from its proper line by an angle of as much as fifteen or more degrees. (See Figs. 43, 46 and 47). From this degree of deformity there are gradations down to a point where the divergence from normal is insignificant in its results. But any material deviation of the great toe has a very appreciable influence upon the strength of the foot—just as no engineer would think of expecting a bridge to have any strength with its trusses bent to form two horizontal planes. In this deformity muscular strength is impaired, as considerable contractile force is wasted where the tendons concerned have to pull around an angle; the foot is shortened, since bending the toe outward decreases the longitudinal radius of the foot, and a certain amount of leverage is thereby lost; finally, the thrust of the foot in moving the body weight is thus made to fall on the inner margin of the toe near its last joint—a region never intended by nature and mechanically unfit to bear this stress—instead of on the planter surface of the last phalanx of the great toe. A foot with marked hallux valgus must hence be considered as abducted and thus as a relatively weak foot. Besides these defects, a foot with considerable hallux valgus usually also presents bunions, corns and ingrowing nails, as the cause which operates to produce the one ultimately tends to produce the others.

The prevention of hallux valgus depends upon the use of a shoe having a sole with a straight inner margin. The remedying of this condition is brought about by the same means, whereby the injurious pressure along the inside of the great toe is removed and the latter is thus given opportunity by a physiological shoe to return toward its normal line. For young men, whose bones are still growing and who have not developed bunions with inflamed joints, much improvement may be expected in the course of some months under the use of the army shoe; but in old soldiers, permanent structural changes in the foot have occurred and no great return toward normal is possible.

The army shoe is not ideal with respect to the straightness of its inner sole margin, but neither was it intended to be. It was not made ideal for the reason that the foot of the average soldier which it was in practice to cover was not perfect in its toe alignment and could not, in the vast majority of cases, be made so.

Where hallux valgus has been long continued, the joints are so weakened, and the anatomical relations of the bones and muscles are so altered, that only very slight pressure is needed to keep the toes in their position of deformity. The tension of too tight or shrunken socks is often quite sufficient to accomplish this, so in attempting to remedy this defect attention must be given to a proper fit of the socks as well as of the shoes.

A condition of valgus or bending of the little toe is not uncommon, and is due to a narrow shoe the outer margin of the sole of which curves inward too greatly. It is of less importance, as the little toe is less concerned than the great toe in the mechanics of marching. The shape of the new army shoe permits of its natural rectification.

Bunions.

These are enlarged bursal sacs over joints, often going on to inflammation. A good example of a bunion is shown in Fig. 47. They ordinarily occur over the second joint of the great toe; less often on the third joint of the little toe. In a general way, the condition may be regarded as an extreme hallux valgus in which the joint also undergoes an often permanent inflammatory alteration. The cause is shoes which are not only too narrow but are built on a pointed last in which both the great and little toes are forced in toward the center of the foot. The latest military shoe is so shaped that it cannot cause bunions (See Fig. 34), and such as are seen in the service have been caused by civilian shoes or by army shoes of an older pattern. Bunions may not only be very painful but they accompany a deformity which anatomically weakens the foot and materially interferes with marching capacity.

Fig. 47

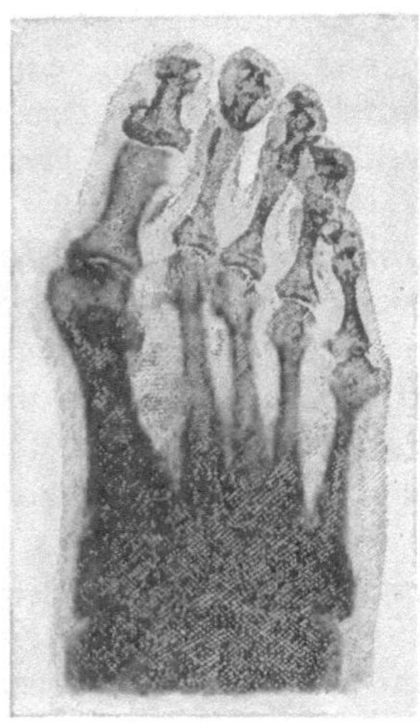

Hallux valgus with bunion and clubbed toes.

In this defect, the phalangeal bone has been pressed out of the straight line which it normally should make with the metatarsal bone with which it articulates—instead of which these two bones meet at an angle, producing inequality of pressure within the joint and causing the bones to tend to absorb at the points of greatest pressure and to build up where pressure is less than normal. This results in alteration of joint structure; while the joint itself, being forced into undue prominence, is forced by the too narrow and mis-shapen shoe into becoming a point of support for the foot and body weight, and constant pressure of the shoe and greater liability to injury sets up inflammation in the bursal sac which, under long use or accidental injury, becomes acute. In such acute inflammation, the skin over the joint becomes red, tense and swollen, while the joint region is excessively very painful on use or under pressure of the shoe upper, and the man is unfitted for marching.

Relatively few bad bunions are found in the service, for if severe they are properly a disqualification for enlistment. A considerable number of small bunions, and a few which are inflamed are, however, found.

In very severe bunions of long standing the only effective treatment is found in a surgical operation requiring removal of bone tissue before the toe can be brought back into proper line. Cases requiring such treatment usually have feet so altered and weakened as to render them unsuitable for military service.

Swollen and inflamed bunions are unfit for marching and should receive the attention of the surgeon.

Ordinary bunions tend to improvement on proper fitting of the feet with the army shoe, since this largely removes pressure from the swollen joint and affords space for the distorted great toe to return toward its proper alignment. The degree of improvement depends upon the size of the bunion, the length of time it has existed, and the age of the patient. Small bunions with young soldiers should give no further trouble with properly fitting army shoes. Large bunions in old soldiers will not greatly improve, since deformity of the bony structure has become permanent; the best that can be expected is to keep them from getting worse and put them under such conditions that they will give no great trouble.

Very large, swollen bunions greatly interfere with proper shoe fitting, for a shoe which does not give painful pressure on the bunion is usually too large for the foot and permits of slippage of the foot in the shoe with great liability to its injury elsewhere. Very large bunions should be cause for discharge of surgeon's certificate of disability. With small ones, the shoes selected should be as loose as can be comfortably worn, and in addition the shoes should be effectively stretched over night with a bunion stretcher, after the leather has been

Fig. 48

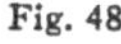

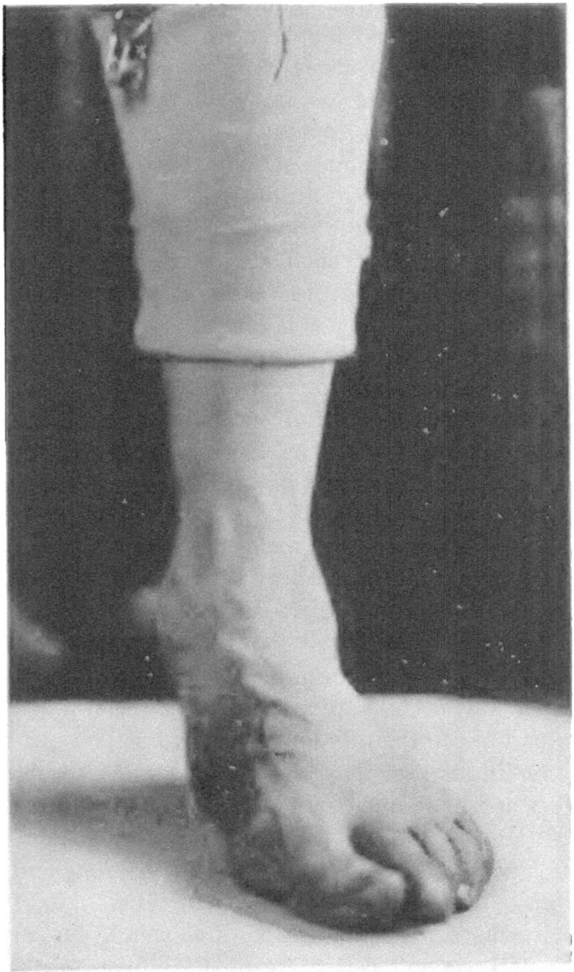

Foot of a soldier, illustrating flat-foot, hallux valgus, clubbed toes, hammer toe.

thoroughly wet, until the shoe shape has been so altered as to take off all pressure over the bunion area.

Rubber spools and springs between the toes, and other patent devices to cause them to spread and return to their proper alignment, are not necessary to the cure of bunions on soldiers' feet—the continued use of the military shoe, and the pressure on the foot and its expansion in marching, should ultimately by themselves bring about good results.

Ingrowing Nails.

This is a condition in which the edges of the nail, curving inward, grow back into the flesh. It usually, but not always, occurs in the great toe. It is often very painful, and the constant irritation frequently results in repeated infections and prolonged suppuration around the matrix of the nail. Such inflammatory attacks incapacitate the soldier from marching.

This condition is caused by shoes which are too narrow across the toes. The particular type of civilian shoe most concerned is that with the socalled "spike toe", in which the great toe is pressed out of its proper alignment and forced toward the center of the foot. But a broader shoe, if the front of the sole is cut away too much on its inner margin, may also cause it; in this latter case, the shoe selected is apt to have been too short, and the nail is pressed back as well as laterally.

Most cases of ingrowing nails are promptly relieved of all symptoms and tend to early cure by the use of a shoe built on a last with a fairly straight inner line and broad across the toes. These requirements are possessed by the army shoe; which latter must also be carefully fitted to the foot as to length and width. The pressure which is the sole cause of the trouble is thus removed, as is shown in Fig. 34.

A small number of ingrowing nails require additional treatment for a few days, consisting of trimming the nail and inserting a pledget of cotton under its offending edge to relieve irritation.

A few cases of ingrowing nails may have gone on to a degree in which surgical treatment, which consists in cutting out a segment of the nail and the matrix from which it grows, is necessary.

Any case of suppuration around a nail, because of the danger of infection which is present, should be sent to see the surgeon.

Clubbed Toes.

This is a condition in which the toes are so compressed as to become bulbous and larger at their ends than along their shafts. It is well shown in Figs. 48 and 49. It is produced by the use of pointed shoes which are too narrow across the toes, though these shoes usually have plenty of vacant space in front of the toes, into which space the latter crowd as a result of pressure behind and then attempt to expand and adjust themselves. The result of this pressure, if continued, is the deviation of the entire toes away from their proper line into a condition of hallux, the compression of the fleshy parts of the shafts of the toes into approximately plane surfaces where they touch each other, and such atrophy of muscles and loss of power in the foot as very greatly tend to produce marching incapacity. Usually it is the second, third and fourth toes which are affected; and a condition is not infrequently seen in which such pressure has resulted in the elongation and projection of the second toe for as much as half an inch in front of the great toe (See Fig. 49). Under such conditions, the toes override and practically become mere fleshy appendages of the foot, the forward thrust of the body in marching practically depending upon the impetus given from the ball of the foot with such assistance as may be possible from a coincidently weakened great toe. With feet deformed in this way, the ends of the smaller toes are often blistered and calloused, the nails are deformed and thickened, a corn usually forms over the last joint of the little toe and a bunion over its metatarso-phalangeal joint, while one or more soft corns, usually of a very painful character, develop between the compressed toes. The skin between the toes, kept soft and moist

Fig. 49

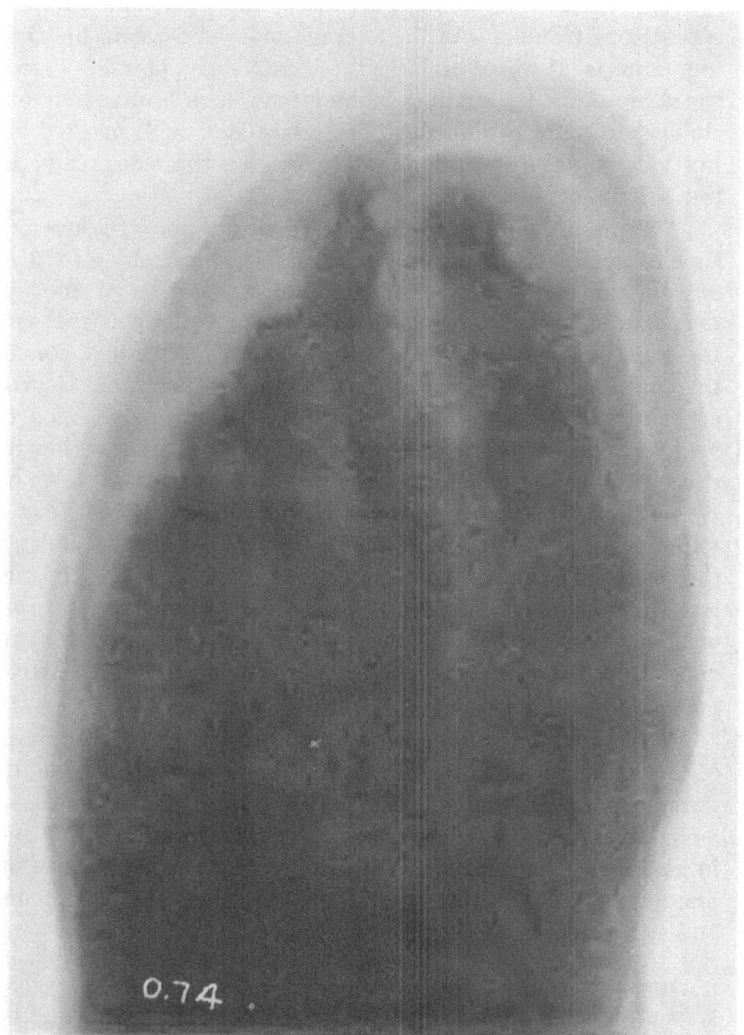

Highly deformed foot of the same soldier shown in Figs. 42 and 48, supporting full weight of field equipment, in new military shoe.

Note the clubbed second toe, hallux valgus and difficulty in fitting which they cause.

by contact, becomes tender, irritated, reddened and prone to eczematous trouble. As the average man who wears his shoes too tight is also apt to select an extremely pointed pattern based more upon prevailing fashion than upon human anatomy, clubbed toes are ordinarily found associated with marked hallux valgus, painful bunions, and corns on the sides, ends and tops of the smaller toes.

The prevention of clubbed toes depends upon the use of a shoe of sufficient breadth and reasonably approaching in shape of sole the conformation of the anterior portion of the normal foot, and improvement and cure depend upon the same factor. The new army shoe is based upon a proper conception of the soldier's foot, and its shape is such that, if properly fitted, it cannot exert any injurious compression upon the toes. (See Fig. 34). Free movement of the latter within this shoe is always possible. By the continued use of such a shoe the feet of the average soldier, deformed in this way, may be expected to return in time materially toward the normal. In the younger class of soldiers the affected toes will in time lose their angular appearance, round out in contour, and their ends diminish in size, while freedom from compression and opportunity for use causes fleshy development and enlargement along the shaft.

In old soldiers with considerable defect of this nature much of the damage is permanent, as the bony framework has undergone definite changes and the overlying soft tissue is of a character that does not permit of great alteration. But even in these cases the army shoe should remove any cause for discomfort, and in time permit of the material development and straightening of the front of the foot.

Hammer Toes.

This is a condition in which the last joint of the toe is permanently flexed at a right angle, so that the tip of the toe strikes the sole of the shoe in walking. The condition is one which unfits for enlistment, as the deformed position of the toe is such that a sensitive bearing surface is created and dirt and grit are apt to work under the nail and produce inflammation. However, some cases slip by recruiting officers, and a few have undoubtedly been developed in the service as a result of the men being allowed to select their own shoes. The second and third toes are the ones usually affected, and these also commonly present corns over their last joints. The condition is generally associated with clubbed toes.

This foot deformity is produced by too short shoes, whereby the toes are pressed back and forced to double up under themselves. If this condition is long continued, the toe assumes a bent position from permanent contraction of the muscles of the sole of the foot. Adhesions may form within the joint and it may lose its function. In the latter case, the soldier should be discharged. The more severe cases should be sent to the surgeon, who may find it desirable to do an operation to lengthen the contracted tendon. Mild cases will greatly improve and may give no further trouble if the soldier is made to wear a shoe long enough and broad enough to permit of the return of the toe to its proper extension and anatomical relation.

Hammer toes are invariably caused by a badly fitting shoe, with an improper shape of the shoe as a minor contributing factor. They cannot be produced in a shoe of the shape of the new military shoe, if the latter is fitted so that a vacant space of approximately half an inch exists between the toe of the shoe and the toe of the foot when expanded under the entire weight of the body and equipment.

Flat-foot.

In true flat-foot the relations of the skeleton of the foot are altered and the bony arch of the foot is more or less completely broken down. (See Figs. 48, 50, 51 and 52). Where it is well developed, this condition is cause for rejection for enlistment, as it is a complete disqualification for marching. Cases may, however, develop in the military service, and especially in newly raised troops, as a result of injudicious marching when the feet are not in proper condition for it. But care must be taken to differentiate between a flat-foot which is real and that which is only apparent, for the negro race presents a foot type the arch of which is flattened from the Caucasian standard and yet does not interfere with marching. So, too, there are white individuals whose foot type is negroid in character. There are also others whose muscular development of the sole is so great as almost to fill up and obliterate the foot arch and whose foot-prints therefore more or less resemble those of flat feet.

In connection with this subject it must be mentioned that the common idea that all pain in the arch of the foot is due to flat-foot is incorrect, and the cause of such pain may be looked for in one of several conditions.

Fig. 50

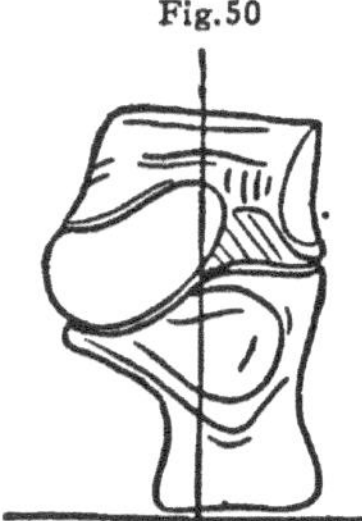

The relation of the astragalus to the os calcis in the normal foot. (Whitman.)

Fig. 51

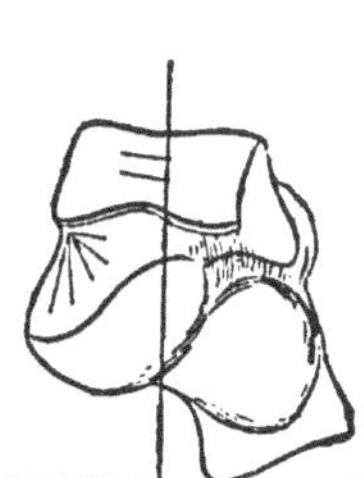

The relation of the astragalus and os calcis in the flat foot. (Whitman.)

True flat-foot presents a foot which, looked at from the side, is flattened over the instep. Looked at from in front, the inner part of the foot appears to be sunken and the inner ankle bone to be unusually prominent, giving the general impression of the foot being everted outward.. (See Figs. 48, 50 and 51). The general impression of the foot is that it is undeveloped and somewhat lengthened. The man will have a clumsy gait, and if the condition has long existed he will be knock kneed or have a marked tendency thereto. He will complain of painful arches on long standing or on marching, and in field equipment will usually break down and fall out after going a very few miles. The condition will be verified by having him step in a basin of water and then walk on a bare floor, or by sending him to the hospital to have the soles of his feet inked and be made to walk over pieces of paper. The footprints in either case will show imprint of the whole or greater part of the foot arch, demonstrating—in connection with the other signs—that the arch has fallen. Fig. 48 shows a case of true flat-foot, and Fig. 52 the footprint of the same soldier. The latter should be compared with Fig. 15, which shows a normal footprint.

But a stocky, muscular foot, with a high instep and thick in vertical section, or which gives no pain in marching, is not true flat-foot even though the footprint, taken by itself, might tend to indicate the contrary. This is an important point, for many soldiers are regarded as having flat-foot who, in fact, do not have it.

The cause of flat-foot is pressure from above, upon structures of a strength inadequate to support it. This pressure may act quite rapidly in producing its results, or it may extend over considerable periods of time and the flat-foot finally produced be of very gradual development. It has already been pointed out, in connection with the anatomy of the foot, that the arch is not a rigid structure but is composed of a number of small bones bound firmly together by ligaments, mostly running from front to rear, and that these ligaments are reinforced by a series of layers of muscles, similarly disposed. Also that the foot arch is a "bow string arch", in which a large part of the arch support is derived from the tension of the muscles attached to its two ends. The arch is further filled up, and is thus in a way buttressed from below, if these foot muscles are well developed and a reasonable amount of fatty tissue is present.

These muscles may be said to be adjusted to bear a certain stress and support a certain weight. In the case of a recruit fresh from civil life, this weight may be considered to be that of the body alone; and any additional weight, as that of the rifle and equipment, brings a strain on the foot muscles which, without their development and training, they are not pre-

Fig. 52

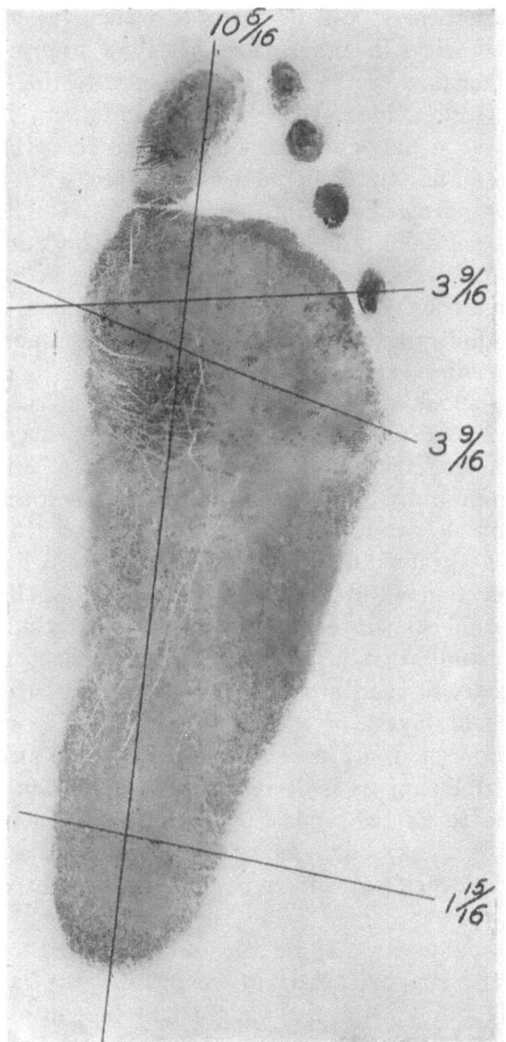

Flat foot. Foot print of the same foot shown in Fig. 48.

pared adequately to support. The muscles then, like elastic bands, stretch under the unaccustomed pressure until a considerable or even the greater part of the strain falls upon the ligaments. If the ligaments are also weak, they too begin to yield under the strain and the arch tends to collapse under the pressure from above. In other words, to prevent flat-foot, muscular tension on the sole of the foot ought exert a force greater than—or at least counterbalance—that of the weight to be borne.

Now, if an untrained recruit—and particularly one in whom a previous sedentary occupation has not resulted in fair foot development—be suddenly made to carry the military burden and undertake a hard march, this physiological balance, as adjusted for different conditions, may be disturbed, and the feet suffer an injury which may be permanent. It is particularly important to remember this fact at recruit depots and in the raising of volunteer troops, when there is every incentive to transform the civilian into the soldier in the shortest possible time—for misdirected energy in this respect may result in promptly spoiling many of what might otherwise be developed into excellent soldiers.

Flat-foot may also develop in soldiers who have had well developed feet, but whose foot muscles have weakened and thinned as a result of prolonged non-use; as, for example, long confinement to hospital with typhoid fever or other wasting disease. Such cases may, in convalescence, rapidly take on body weight without compensating muscular development, and to take such men off sick report so that they can accompany their organizations on a march is to subject them to the same risks—or even greater ones—as attend the marching of recruits under such conditions.

Or flat-foot may result from the stretching of the muscles, due to their fatigue from over marching or long standing.

Also wearing shoes with too high heels causes flat-foot, since the more the heel is raised above the ground by the shoe the more the weight of the body and burden is shifted toward the front part of the foot arch, which is weaker and less adapted to resist pressure.

Another point is that where the shoe is too narrow and the toes are compressed, and especially where this is combined with a faulty shape of the shoe producing hallux valgus, the normal support of the body is altered. To better maintain its equilibrium under such conditions, the toes must be turned out in an exaggerated position of "attention" in standing, and in marching the man tends to walk splay-footed. (See Fig. 23). In both instances, the weight of the body falls directly on the inner part of the ankle joint, and over the arch of the foot at its weakest point. This directly tends—especially in persons with undeveloped feet, those recovering from prolonged illness and those untrained to carry heavy burdens—to cause the foot arch to spread and produce flat-foot.

In bare feet, or in sufficiently broad, low-heeled shoes, however, the toe tends to point directly forward, or even inward, in walking, as in the case of the naked savage, non-shoe wearing child or moccasined Indian, (see Figs. 19 and 22) in which classes flat-foot rarely if ever occurs. Here the adducted great toe supports the anterior inner pillar of the foot arch and keeps the foot from rolling inwards. This position throws the body weight on the outer part of the ankle, away from the arch and directly over a part of the foot intended to support weight and which lies everywhere in direct contact with the ground for that purpose. (See Fig. 5). Narrow, pointed shoes thus greatly favor flat-foot; broad physiological shoes materially tend to prevent it in spite of the opposite impression of the wearer, unaccustomed to broad shoes, that his foot is breaking down. The truth of this contention can be verified by any one by standing with the feet in the position of "attention", and then with the heels and toes of the two feet in contact, or at least parallel.

The prevention of flat-foot therefore resolves itself into three considerations; first, that a weak foot shall not be overloaded or overtaxed; second, that the weak foot shall be so strengthened as to be able to support any military burden, under any military conditions, without injury; third, that the shoe worn shall be broad and sensible.

The first merely implies the exercise of ordinary common sense in not letting the recruit with any tendency to weak feet, or the recently debilitated, carry the full equipment over long distances until after a suitable course of training.

The second requirement implies development of foot strength in such men by a course of training which includes much marching with gradual progressive increase in the distance to be marched, and weight of the equipment to be carried, until the maximum of both is reached.

For men with apparent tendency to breaking down of the foot arch, special foot exercises, particularly intended to develop the muscles of the sole of the foot, should be carried out in addition to practice in marching. These foot exercises include:

(a) Rising high on the toes; then slowly lowering the body until the heel rests on the ground; then repeating the above movements. Probably five minutes of this, both morning and night, will be sufficient. In this exercise, the man must rise as high as possible on his toes; since in rising only part way the muscles of the calf are chiefly concerned and not those of the foot which it is desired to develop.

(b) Climbing up and down flights of stairs is good exercise to strengthen the foot muscles.

(c) An excellent exercise is to have the man sit in a chair, shoes off. Resting his heel against the floor, he forcibly bends and inverts the foot. This exercise can be made much more severe in the gymnasium or barracks by hooking the toes over the handle of a light chest weight or exerciser.

All these special exercises should be continued and progressively increased until the muscles concerned feel quite tired. Usually exercising from five to seven minutes twice daily is long enough at the outset. The special exercises will need to be continued for several weeks, the time necessarily depending on the degree of foot defect and the rapidity with which it is corrected. The man should endeavor to keep his toes turned to the front in marching.

Above all things, patent devices intended to support the foot arch should be avoided by soldiers with a tendency to weak or flat feet. These arch supports may give a sensation of relief when worn, but they relieve the symptom of discomfort at the expense of making the underlying cause of the latter much worse, for they splint and restrict the use of the very muscles upon the development and strengthening of which the regaining and preservation of the foot arch depends. Such arch supports are impossible of use in military marching, and once habituated to them, the wearer's feet are so much weakened that he is helpless without them.

For weak arches, and threatened flat feet, a "valgus wedge" may be of service and will do no harm as a temporary corrective. This consists in raising the inner border of the sole and heel by a piece of leather one-eighth of an inch thick at its inner aspect and getting thinner as it gets nearer the center. This throws the weight away from the foot arch on to the outer border of the foot and also causes the toes to be pointed more to the front in walking. As the muscles strengthen, the leather strips are reduced in thickness until the normal sole and heel are reached.

Severe cases of flat feet should be discharged from the service. While their condition can undoubtedly be improved, the prospects of complete return to a foot arch suitable for marching are too doubtful to make worth while the expenditure of the time and effort which must necessarily be involved.

Since many recruits are enlisted who have weak feet, and since the tendency of much early military training is to result in the excessive use of such feet unprepared to stand any severe strain, it would seem desirable for organization commanders to lay special stress on foot exercises for these men new to the service. Many gymnasia have foot exercising apparatus, which at present are not properly utilized.

Painful Arches.

This condition is found in flat feet and also those in which there is beginning breaking down. It is also found in feet with perfectly normal arches but in which the sole muscles are weak, either from lack of development or atrophy due to sickness, or in which they are not yet adapted to the increased strain due to carrying an unaccustomed burden. Further, perfectly normal and strongly developed feet, when put into broader and looser shoes than those to which they are habituated, develop pain and the sensation of breaking down on marching—due to the stretching of muscles and ligaments beyond the limits to which they were accustomed, under the forcible foot expansion resulting from marching and burden carrying. This is particularly true of those who have been wearing shoes built on crooked or pointed lasts, in which the foot is accustomed to support from the fixed point provided by the back of the shoe in the rear and similar points in front on the inner aspect of the great toe, and outer aspect of the little toe, caused by the forcing of these toes toward the center and into a space too narrow for the foot.

The pain, of an aching character, is usually referred to the region of the high instep and extends through the foot to the sole under the foot arch. It will be present in greater or less degree in probably a majority of soldiers who have been fitted with the broad army shoe and then shortly afterward given hard marching under field equipment. Ordinarily, such pain signifies nothing and wears away in a very few days as soon as the foot muscles and ligaments stretch and adapt themselves to the new conditions of greater foot expansion. Sometimes lowering the heel by taking off one thickness of leather will give relief, as the center of gravity is thus shifted nearer the heel and less weight is thereby thrown on the weaker fore-foot.

Whenever arch pain persists over a week or more, it is well to give the foot a careful examination, as it may be that the arch is really breaking down in the production of true flatfoot or that teno-synovitis is present.

Recruits, newly enlisted volunteers, and militia wearing the army shoe only occasionally, will be the ones chiefly liable to painful arches of this character.

Fracture of Metatarsals.

This injury is not common in our army. In the German army, with its heavy, clumsy footwear, it is said to cause from 20 to 40 admissions to sick report out of each 1,000 admissions. It is most common in young soldiers, and apparently is the result of sudden jar from stepping on a stone or inequality in the road, especially with a sole which has worn thin. The most frequent location of the fracture is the head of the 2nd, 3rd or 4th metatarsal bone. The diagnosis can rarely be made with certainty without the use of the X-ray. The injury of course incapacitates for marching.

Painful Heel.

This condition has no visible signs and its cause is not well understood. It is not uncommon in persons who are much on their feet, as policemen and letter carriers, and may be found among soldiers. It seems to be due to slight but continued bruising of the heel from repeated impact against a possibly unfitting surface. Such cases can usually be relieved by wearing heavy wool socks, by having rubber heels put on their shoes, or by very cautiously cutting out a little of the calfskin heel lining immediately under the painful area, taking pains to carefully smooth off the cut edges. Sometimes a slight loosening or wrinkling of the sock lining of the heel of the shoe is at fault, and this possibility should be investigated.

Anterior Metatarsalgia.

This is a painful condition usually referred to the joint at the base of the fourth toe. It is not common in the service, and would be looked for chiefly in recruits and officers rather than old soldiers. It is often associated with a depressed arch and in feet with relatively little muscular development. There is usually a painful callous on the ball beneath the affected joint. The cause is not definitely known; but a shoe in which there is too much "spring"—in which the toes are turned up by a sole with too much curve—and in which there is a lowering of the insole in the center with raising of the lateral edges to form a shallow trough in which the heads of the interior metatarsal bones are jammed together in standing or walking, seems to be largely at fault. If shoes wear away in the center, the sinking of the sole makes a concavity into which the ball of the foot sinks and becomes more or less convex and compressed toward the center. The pain is peculiar in that it is spasmodic, and usually comes on and subsides suddenly. It may come on after the march is over, or even during the sleeping hours. The pain often begins as a tingling, burning sensation. The cases should usually be sent to see the surgeon. Prevention and treatment are found in the use of shoes with broad, flat soles, and in the measures recommended for strengthening the muscles and arch of the foot.

Teno-Synovitis.

This is a painful, inflammatory condition of muscle tendons, due to an injury of some sort. The tendons so affected usually lie close to the surface. In the foot, those most liable to injury lie on the top over the instep, where protective fat, muscle or other tissue is scanty and the tendons are liable to injury from blows or from pressure between the shoe above and the hard, unyielding bone below. The tendon most liable to this injury is the one running across the instep and especially concerned in lifting the great toe. The pain is apt to come on after hard marching and often in soldiers who have previously had no foot trouble. It may be referred to the foot arch and may at first arouse suspicion of weak arches. There is, however, no flattening of the feet, and the latter are usually strong and well developed. The foot presents no physical change of appearance, but there is tenderness on touch along part or nearly all of the tendon concerned. Sometimes a grating sensation may be felt along the course of the tendon affected. A little rest usually puts the feet in good condition again, but some cases last longer. The cause is probably usually due to too tight lacing, with unnecessarily severe pressure on the tendons below. A knot in the shoe lace may cause it. The relatively small number of eyelets in the military shoe may perhaps favor it, as not equally distributing pressure across the foot but causing it to become greater than is desirable at the several points crossed by, and immediately under, the shoe laces. Prevention consists in lacing the shoe tightly enough to keep it firmly in position, but not so tight as to work an injury to the foot structures lying below. The shoe lace used should be broad and flat, and attention given to preventing it from rolling into a cord with use. The relief of pressure on painful areas, by suitably adjusted strips of blanket inserted between the tongue and lacing, should be of much value. Frequent bathing the foot in cold water is useful as both a preventive as well as curative measure.

Blisters and Abrasions.

These are usually caused by friction, less often by impact, and in some few instances by pressure. In a blister, the irritation causes a local flow and collection of serum between the inner and outer layers of the skin, lifting up the latter. The size of the blister depends on the area of the skin sufficiently irritated to result in such outward evidence of injury. Some may be very large, especially those of the heel. The locality of blisters depends upon the particular divergence of the shoe from the shape of the foot it is intended to cover. Thus the same shoe might cause different injuries in two feet of the same size but different conformation. Blisters are painful, as the serum which has flowed into the local tissues causes pressure and irritation of the sensitive nerve filaments. This pain is greatly increased by continuation of the rubbing or striking which caused the blister in the first place, and may very frequently become so great as to incapacitate the sufferer from marching. Blisters are also liable to become infected, and in such cases may become the starting point from which the deeper structures of the foot and leg subsequently become dangerously infected and perhaps loss of limb or even life results.

The prevention and cure of blisters implies the avoidance or removal of their cause. Their presence is evidence of either locally ill fitting shoes, or of areas as yet untoughened by lack of sufficient previous contact with an opposing surface. Treatment of blisters thus includes measures directed to both the shoe and foot. The cause, whatever it be, must be sought out and removed. For instance, the shoe may be generally too large, which defect can perhaps be largely corrected by the wearing of two pairs of socks; more snug lacing may be necessary to prevent recurrence of a heel blister; a blister on the outside of the little toe may call for the use of the shoe stretcher over that area; a blister over the top of the base of the great toe might be due to a hard wrinkle in the leather, due to wetting, which should have been softened and oiled after drying, etc., etc. So long as the exciting cause remains unremedied, blisters will tend to recur.

Blisters are treated by pricking them with a clean needle and gently pressing out their contents. Under no circumstances should the raised cuticle be torn away. The blister proper, and any reddened area around it, is then covered with a piece of zinc oxide plaster, as supplied by the Medical Department. This plaster does not stick well to a moist skin, so the latter should be wiped dry; the plaster also does not stick well unless applied hot, so a match is burned close to the adhesive surface until the latter shows small, sticky bubbles. The plaster is then pressed down smoothly over the blister, where the raised epidermis usually soon grows back in position. Ordinarily the soldier can continue marching, under protection of the plaster, without pain, and recovery is complete in a couple of days; as in many instances only a slight amount of protection to the affected area is necessary and a little immobilization and relief from friction is all that is required. It has frequently been seen where a soldier, whose shoes were bad fits, completed a march of several days without difficulty though his feet ultimately had to be largely covered with such plaster strips.

In a few instances, however, the blister becomes infected and, instead of healing, goes on to suppuration. This is indicated by plain, puffiness and redness in the vicinity of the blister. The presence of suppuration may be determined by gently raising one edge of the plaster when, if pus be present, it can be pressed out. If suppuration exists, the man should see the surgeon without delay and have the abrasion disinfected and dressed.

Abrasions are simply blisters from which the cuticle forming the outer wall has been torn off. They are very painful from access of the air and material of the sock to the bared nerve filaments and thus readily incapacitate for marching. They are always infected, but small superficial abrasions usually readily heal under the zinc oxide plaster, which is itself mildly germicidal.

The large abrasions would usually suppurate under plaster; and such cases should see the surgeon, who will ordinarily cause a disinfectant solution and gauze dressing to be applied.

If zinc oxide plaster be not available, the blister may be evacuated, greased and pressed back into position, where atmospheric pressure tends to hold it. Often two or three turns of a light bandage over the blister may be used in the shoe, and at night its bandaging is of course practicable. But where bandaging is employed, care should be taken lest the thickness of the protective material applied over the affected area increase the already excessive pressure over that part. To apply a wad of anything, as cloth or cotton, over a blister will certainly make it worse.

Painting abrasions with a five or ten per cent solution of chromic acid is a treatment used in the French and German armies. A five per cent solution of picric acid, such as is used in treating burns, may also be employed in the treatment of ordinary abrasions; in fact, the manner in which cuticle is raised and lost in blisters and abrasions is much like that in burns of the first degree.

In a general way, it may be said that blisters and abrasions, callosities and corns indicate the existence of harmful pressure by a shoe which is too small over the area in which these blemishes occur. These points of irritation, if sought for, can always be found and appropriate measures for removal can usually be carried out with more or less complete success.

But also occasionally a shoe which is too large over the region of the blemish permits the occurrence of an injurious friction which is the cause of the trouble. This local excess in size may, however, have its cause in an attempt to relieve the foot from pressure elsewhere. Such a cause was common in former army shoes which were too low over the instep, whereby the soldier in order to get a shoe high enough for his instep was forced to take a shoe too long for his foot and too large for his heel.

In determining a cause for the above foot blemishes, it is thus necessary to give due consideration to the two apparently dissimilar factors of tightness and looseness.

Blisters on top of the toes are usually due to pressure from the toe cap being too low or too stiff. The judicious use of the shoe stretcher may remove this condition, though what is probably needed is a larger shoe. Blisters on the ends of the toes are evidence that the shoe is too short or that it was not sufficiently tightly laced—in either case the remedy suggests itself. Blisters on the sides of the little or big toe usually indicate that the shoe is too narrow; the remedy being either use of the shoe stretcher or a greater width. Foot blisters sometimes occur along the marginal lines where the outer and inner aspects of the foot come in contact with the shoe insole. These are usually due to defect of construction causing a poor fit between the shoe insole and upper, by which one or both sides of the foot extend over an open space between the insole and upper, forming an inequality in the shoe surface on which the foot bears. Similarly, ridges may be present in these regions, due to the insole curling up along its edges as a result of wetting and subsequent shrinking and warping. The first condition is due to careless manuacture and inspection of the shoe, and is perhaps best met by the soldier by the use of heavier socks. The second is due to either poor material, bad workmanship or lack of care of the shoe. The best remedy is to adjust the shoe on an iron last so that the latter comes in contact with all parts of the offending ridges, and pound the latter down flat with a hammer.

Heel blisters are due to a shoe not being properly laced up or to a bad sock. The remedies for these are obvious. They are also due to shoes being too long, or not fitting sufficiently snugly over the instep and around the ankle. Better selection, or the use of a cloth pad under the lacing, will prevent bad results from these conditions.

Fig. 53

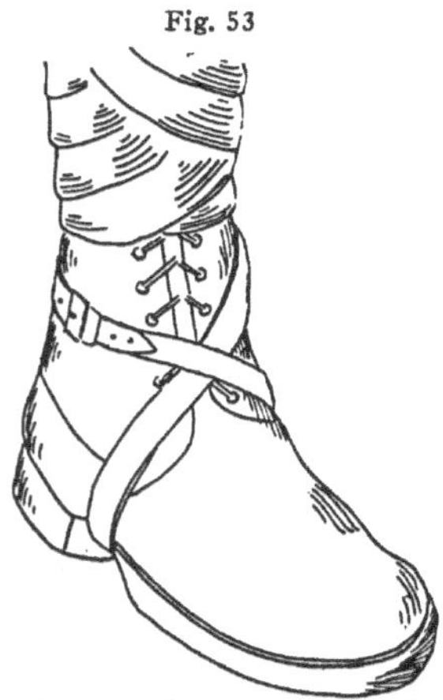

Marching strap of the French Army. (From Journal of the Royal Army Medical Corps.)

With the few men whose large feet and slender ankles render shoe fitting difficult, and who are thus obliged to use somewhat too loose shoes in marching, the French army marching strap (See Fig. 53) may be used to give a more snug fit over the instep and above the heel and prevent the shoe from slipping up and down and chafing the back of the foot. In the absence of a strap, any suitable material capable of producing sufficient tension may be used for this purpose.

Blisters and callosities develop over the bottom of the sole or heel from inequalities due to various causes. One of these may be warping of the sole of the shoe in drying after wetting, in which case little can be done in the way of remedy except the use of heavier socks and efforts to hammer the sole—after wetting—flat on an iron last; if these measures are unsatisfactory the shoes should be discarded. Another cause is the wearing of socks with holes or darns, the remedy for which is obvious. Again, a sock may wrinkle into a fold during the march, or gravel or sand work into the shoe; under such conditions the man should pull his sock tight or take off and clean out his shoe at the next hourly halt, or be encouraged to fall out and do this at once on the march if the discomfort is more than trifling. Corns also form on the ball of the foot through unduly high heels throwing the weight too much forward and bringing excessive pressure over this point.

Blisters are often caused by tender feet, the skin of which is untoughened and unaccustomed to withstand friction and pressure as a result of lack of practice in marching. Areas of skin of this nature are brought into hurtful contact with the sole when narrow shoes are exchanged for wider ones and the bottom of the foot is thus allowed fully to flatten out. Too narrow shoes also cause foot blisters, as they compress the sole into ridges upon which the wearer of such shoes is constantly walking.

The soldier is expected to have two pairs of serviceable shoes with him in the field at all times. It is desirable to have these shoes alternated in use day by day. Even though these shoes be of the same last and be stamped with an identical size and letter, and thus supposedly the same, still they will not feel exactly the same to the foot. The reason is that the bulk of lasts varies slightly with variation in atmospheric moisture; leather cut from different skins, or parts of the same skin, stretches unequally; and shoes pulled from the lasts earlier shrink more than shoes left on longer. It thus happens that exchange of shoes apparently identical may give relief to sore places by transference of painful pressure to other less sensitive parts.

Corns.

These are localized callosities of the skin of the foot resulting from continued injury by ill fitting shoes. They have their starting point in a blister or abrasion, in the repair of which nature guards against repetition of such injury by thickening the skin with a stouter, harder horny layer. If the local irritation and injury continues, whether from chafing, pressure or impact, the outer layer of the skin continues to thicken locally until its sufficiency for protective purposes is exceeded; while pressure of this horn-like layer, and its root-like prolongations extending deeper into the flesh, cause much pain in the little nerves lying underneath. This pain may be very considerable, and quite sufficient to very materially diminish or even destroy marching capacity.

The cause of corns is found in badly fitting shoes, either those being worn at present or which have been worn at some time in the past. In the army, the latter is more usually the case, and a fair proportion of the corns noted in soldiers are inheritances from the use of the mis-shapen civilian styles of shoes worn before enlistment. In determining the matter of the prevention and treatment of corns in any given individual, the question of whether the cause still remains or is no longer existent needs always to be determined in relation to both treatment and cure. If it remains, it must be removed, either by judicious use of the shoe stretcher in the removal of local pressure, or by at once discarding such shoes as are not susceptible of suitable improvement. It is useless to expect to cure corns while their cause is permitted to remain.

Constant attention to corns will largely bring relief from the pain and annoyance which they cause. External corns, after softening by soaking the foot in warm soap suds, may be carefully pared down several times a month—but great care should be taken not to draw blood in cutting down the corn, as these little wounds in this region are apt to become dangerously infected and have not rarely caused serious illness and death. If such a little injury is inflicted, it is usually sufficient to wash away the blood and smear a very little corn salve or corn collodion on the wound, or cover it well with foot powder and a bit of zinc oxide plaster or clean cloth. But cutting corns brings only temporary relief and does not cure the trouble. Soft corns, which are those located between the toes, cannot well be thus trimmed or pared. They require the application of medicine to kill and soften the corn tissue, so that the latter may readily come away without pain. The following combinations are very effective in assisting in the removal of both soft and hard corns and callouses:

Corn Collodion.

Salicylic Acid	11 parts
Extract of Cannabis Indica	2 parts
Alcohol	10 parts
Flexible collodion, enough to make a total of 100 parts	

The materials for the above are supplied by the Medical Department. If necessary, the cannabis indica may be left out. The solution is inflammable and should be kept away from lighted matches, cigars, cigarettes, etc. It evaporates rapidly if open to the air, and hence the bottle should be kept tightly corked except when directly in use. No great amount of the solution is needed, and a small bottle of about one ounce should be enough to treat a couple of dozen cases. To apply it, a bit of cotton is twisted around the end of a match or splinter, dipped in the solution, and used to mop off the corn and the skin in its immediate vicinity.

Another excellent corn medicine is composed as follows:

Corn Salve.

Salicylic Acid	40 parts
Vaseline	30 parts
Lanolin	30 parts

This makes a fairly stiff ointment. For soft corns, it is simply smeared over the corn between the toes. In hard external corns and callouses, it is smeared over the corn and for about an eighth of an inch beyond the margin of the latter, and the whole is covered and kept from being wiped off by a strip of zinc oxide plaster.

Commercial corn plasters are usually merely felt rings which are made to adhere to the skin around the corn and give comfort by removing painful pressure. One or two brands are medicated so that while giving relief from pain they assist in the removal of the corn. They are not supplied by the Medical Department and have no greater merit than the corn salve and corn collodion already mentioned.

The best way to remove corns is as follows:

1. (a) Wash the foot thoroughly at bed time; then soak

it for at least ten minutes in hot soap suds. The corn then becomes soft to the touch and whitish in appearance.

(b) Wipe the foot and corn dry.

(c) Paint the entire corn, and for at least an eighth of an inch around it, with several coats of the corn collodion already mentioned, and let it dry.

Or apply the corn salve, covering the corn and salve with zinc oxide plaster.

2. Repeat the procedure given in (a), (b) and (c) on the following night; previously removing any plaster from the foot.

3. Repeat the procedure given in (a), (b) and (c) again the following night.

4. On the fourth night the corn should present a dead, whitish appearance after washing the foot.

Now take the back of the point of a knife and slide it under the loosened dead skin around the margin of the corn. Work around the corn, prying it loose from the foot but taking great care not to cut its attachments and prolongations into the flesh. In this way, a corn may be lifted entire out of its position and a cure at once follow; but if the attachments of the corn are cut through and not pulled out, return of the corn is almost certain to occur. The object is to pull away in one piece all the thickened tissue down to the "quick", but without causing bleeding. If cut away piecemeal, the corn will probably return.

In very large corns with much hard tissue, it may be necessary to continue the treatment given in (a), (b) and (c) for more than three nights. Occasionally five or six nights are necessary. Sometimes it is well to pare away a very thick corn or callous, so that the medicine can strike into the roots better. No effort should be made to take out the corn until it appears dead and peels off from the foot with little difficulty.

If it appears that the corn has not been completely removed, treatment should be renewed in a few days. To do it immediately may make the foot sore. Sometimes several treatments are necessary to get rid of a corn.

This treatment is not of itself painful, but it hardens the corn and thus makes it more uncomfortable until removed. On pulling the corn away, it leaves a bared area which is somewhat sensitive for about a day. For these reasons, the removal of corns should be accomplished prior to, rather than during, a march.

Callouses, wherever located, are treated like corns. Very large ones, which usually occur under the ball of the foot, are sometimes best removed by the surgeon's knife. But men with feet as badly calloused as this are usually unfit to be soldiers.

No corn can be permanently cured if the causes which first produced it are allowed to continue. The latter must be remedied at the time the corn is removed, or a new corn will soon be produced. A shoe which once produced a corn should be discarded, unless it can be stretched as to no longer press or chafe the former corn area.

Sweaty Feet.

There is a condition of the feet, known as bromidrosis or sweaty or stinking feet, which is quite common among soldiers. In this condition the feet sweat profusely, and the secretion rapidly decomposes and is very foul smelling and offensive. The skin of the feet so affected, especially on the soles and between the toes, becomes soft, whitish and dead looking, like that on a washerwoman's hands. It rubs off easily, and blisters and abrasions are apt to form. The affected area often assumes a mottled appearance, and in old severe cases it is reddish, congested and angry looking. An eczematous condition is not infrequently present.

A soldier with this condition is very liable to break down from foot injury in the field, and in garrison he is a nuisance to the unfortunate co-sharers of his squad room. Frequent washing of the feet only temporarily removes the stinking secretions and does not reach their cause.

The treatment is simple and is usually effective. The feet are bathed and carefully dried. The whole affected area is then carefully painted over with a cotton swab dipped in the following solution:

Commercial Formalin (40% solution of Formaldehyde) 10 parts
Water ....90 parts

This solution is allowed to dry on. If the feet begin to burn, the excess of the solution is washed off. Care must be taken to keep it out of fissures and abrasions, or much pain will be caused. The treatment hardens and practically tans the superficial layers of the skin, and reduces the amount and alters the character of the secretions of the offending sweat glands. Applications are usually made every other day, and half a dozen applications usually suffice to cause a cure.

During the treatment, the feet are washed twice daily, the official foot powder furnished by the Medical Department is very freely used, and clean socks are worn.

Other treatments for this condition are the use of potassium permanganate solution, 1-1000 strength, in which the feet are soaked daily. Sometimes finely powdered alum is dusted into the socks.

In the British army, the soldier with sweaty feet is sent to hospital with his footwear for 24 hours. The socks are soaked an hour in 1-2000 bichloride of mercury solution, then rinsed and washed. The shoes are painted inside with a 10% solution of salicylic acid in alcohol. The feet are washed, dried, painted with the same solution and put in clean socks. The whole process with respect to the foot and shoe, which is really their thorough disinfection, is repeated on the following morning.

Fissures.

In a few instances, men will show cracks or fissures of the skin between the toes and in the folds of the skin of the latter. These fissures are usually quite painful, and sometimes tend to bleed readily. They are usually caused as a result of unaccustomed tension of the skin following the putting of men with compressed and contracted feet into broad sensible shoes allowing the normal foot expansion. This condition is usually temporary, and dusting with foot powder suffices; but sometimes touching the fissures with silver nitrate stick hastens recovery.

There is another form of fissure seen in an eczematous condition of the feet. The cure depends on the cure of the eczema, and the man should be sent to see the surgeon.

The Toe Nails.

The toe nails should be trimmed every ten days or two weeks. They should be cut squarely across, as to cut them away around the corners favors ingrowth of the nails. Misshapen and clubbed nails, if very thick, should be pared down.

When the shoes are too short and the toes are doubled back on themselves, or where the toe cap is so low as to press upon the top of the toe, bruises around and under the nail are very liable to occur. Large blood blisters may make their appearance under the nails, which after some weeks drop off, leaving a new nail which is usually rough, thickened and distorted.

Cleanliness of the Feet.

The maintenance of a reasonable degree of cleanliness is the first and most important factor in the care of the feet. Without it, the skin of the feet tends materially to break down, with the formation of blisters and abrasions, in the presence of an irritating combination of dirt, dead epithelium, sebaceous secretion and sweat; these latter substances undergoing an offensive putrefaction through the action of the hurtful bacteria which thrive in such material.

This necessary cleanliness can be accomplished by means of a daily foot bath, in which the foot is thoroughly washed with tepid water and a little mild soap. No great amount of water is necessary for this purpose. In the field, streams or bodies of water are usually available for this purpose; but a canteen full of water, poured on a poncho which has been spread over a slight depression scraped in the ground and thereby forms a watertight foot bath, is quite sufficient. In the absence of even that amount of water, quite good results can be obtained by thoroughly wiping off the foot, especially between the toes, with a wet handkerchief or the end of a towel moistened with a few spoonfuls of water.

It is probably better, in the field, not to use warm water for foot baths. Cool water seems better to allay the sensation of heat and irritation of the feet resulting from their forcible impact on the road for the many thousands of times required in even an ordinary day's march. Cool water does not seem to soften the skin as much as does hot water, which latter effect is undesirable. For the latter reason, no more soap than is necessary to cleanse the feet should be used. After washing, the feet should be carefully dried.

Generally speaking, troops in the field should wash their feet and change their socks as soon as possible after arriving in camp; they may have no opportunity later.

Use of Foot Powder.

The foot powder supplied by the Medical Department has the following formula:

Salicylic Acid	3 parts
Powdered Starch	10 parts
Powdered Talcum	87 parts

This powder is mildly antiseptic and thus healing and deodorant; it exerts a somewhat astringent and drying influence, while it produces a slippery surface of the skin less liable to chafe against the sock. It comes in half pound cans, with sprinkler tops, for garrison use; and in similar quarter pound cans for field use. In garrison, one of these cans should be in every squad room, and in the field there should be two to each platoon.

No great amount of this powder is required at one time, but the whole surface of the foot should be lightly dusted over, with a greater amount sifted in between the toes.

It should be applied immediately after the feet have been washed, dried and received any other attention necessary.

CHAPTER VII.

THE SOCK.

No discussion of the care of the feet is complete without some consideration of the sock, of which the Quartermaster's Department furnishes three kinds.

Of these, one is made of cotton with linen heels and toes. This sock is thin and has little substance and does not furnish much of a cushion for the foot; its non-conducting material and tight, smooth weave are such as not to conduct perspiration readily away from the skin, which is thus kept moist; unless an excellent fit, it tends, especially when damp, to roll into hard wrinkles which shortly produce blisters. This sock is quite comfortable during warm weather. It may be safely used for light duty, but is unsuitable for use in marching by the average man.

The light wool sock supplied to the soldier is woven of equal parts of wool and cotton. Its substance is about twice that of the cotton sock, while its looser mesh and softer material renders it more comfortable to the foot than the former. Perspiration is readily taken up from the skin and transmitted by its fibres to the outside of the sock where it is more readily evaporated. In marching, it tends to stretch and accommodate itself to the foot rather than to roll into wrinkles. For the average man, it is the best sock to use in marching in all weather except that well below freezing. But there are a few soldiers, especially those with sweaty feet, who claim that the wool in it irritates their skin and makes them uncomfortable. This sock, rather than the cotton one, should habitually be worn when shoes are fitted, so as to make sure that a sufficiently large size suitable for marching is secured.

The quartermaster's heavy woolen sock is made of pure wool. It has all the virtues of the light wool sock, but is too warm for the use of the average man in hot weather, though very excellent during cold, stormy weather. However, not a few old soldiers prefer to use this sock for marching at all times. Its bulk within the shoe is about twice that of the light wool sock, which fact must be taken into account in fitting shoes for use in cold weather. Ordinarily, an increased allowance of about a half size in length and two letters in width will be needed when this sock is to be worn.

Whatever be the kind of sock selected for use, it is of essential importance that it should fit the wearer. If too large, it forms folds which are certain to cause blisters and abrasions. If too small, it is not only uncomfortable but causes tension on the toes which presses them together out of their proper alignment and has a constant tendency to produce hallux valgus, clubbed toes and ingrowing nails. With men whose feet have been deformed and weakened by bad shoes, the tension of too small socks can press them into improper shape almost as badly as ill fitting shoes. The thicker the sock, the greater the tension which it can exert on an enclosed foot; hence the special importance of carefully fitting the thicker wool socks which should be used in marching. Moreover, if the sock be too small, the tension favors rapid wearing through, especially on the heel and toes.

There are five sizes of socks issued, viz. from 9½ to 11½. The addition of a size 12 would be desirable. The size marked on the sock indicates its foot length in inches when the sock is new and is flattened laterally from heel to toe. The cubic capacity of the sock is based on the average foot in civil life. But the soldier's foot is broader and more muscular, and the stocking to be selected for him must usually allow for slight stretching as to width by a little apparent excess as to length. Hence a man with a foot 10½ inches in length will usually require a size 11 sock. But the sock, unlike the shoe, is not a rigid foot covering but is capable of some expansion and very considerable contraction. All socks tend to shrink on washing; this is not great with the cotton sock, but is very considerable in socks of part or all wool, and especially where the latter are subjected to considerable rubbing, and particularly to boiling, in the process of washing. Thus a sock quite large enough for the wearer when drawn may ultimately so contract in size as to become unfit for his use in marching. For this reason, an originally good measurement cannot be depended upon to furnish a permanently good fit in a marching sock.

The use of socks with holes, or darned socks, should be strictly prohibited in marching. Both are extremely liable to produce blisters and abrasions. Even an apparent trifling defect in the sock, especially over the heel, may cause serious foot trouble.

It has been advised to rub the inside of the sock with soap before marching; this undoubtedly reduces friction and its dangers, but the alkali in the soap softens the outer layer of the skin and tends to cause it to break down much more readily.

Some soldiers grease their socks, or accomplish the same result by rubbing the feet with a candle, unsalted beef fat or vaseline. There is no objection to this practice, which undoubtedly reduces friction and the corresponding liability to foot injury.

But the best thing to use for this purpose is the regulation foot powder, of which, after the foot has been well dusted, a little may be sprinkled into the sock itself. This powder not only reduces friction, but also exerts a disinfectant, preservative and curative action on the skin.

It is absolutely necessary that the socks used in marching be clean. Nothing more conduces to tender feet than do dirty socks, in the filth and sweat of which hurtful bacteria multiply rapidly. On the march, a clean pair of socks must be put on daily. The best time for this is of course after the soldier washes his feet on reaching camp. At least one extra pair of good socks must be carried on the soldier's person in the field, and two pairs would be better. As they are light, the extra weight to be carried is a matter of no significance.

Ordinarily, the soldier, after washing his feet, should at once wash the socks he has taken off. Only a cupful of water, if the latter be scarce, is necessary for this purpose, improvising a wash basin from the poncho as described under cleanliness of the feet. After washing, and rinsing out any remaining soap, the socks are dried in the sun, before the fire or by hanging up during the night. In the morning they are dry and ready to go in the pack for use at the day's camp.

If socks cannot be washed, they can at least be changed, the dirty socks dried in the sun and thoroughly beaten and worked with the hands to remove dirt and hardness before being put back in the pack. This very materially assists in their purification and renders them less irritating to the feet when next worn.

Some part of the sock will always be in contact with the same part of the shoe, and the areas thus exposed to friction are the first to wear through. Shoes which are too loose tend to wear out socks rapidly. Changing socks from one foot to another, by creating new areas of contact, will delay their wearing out.

The life of a good fitting light wool sock, in a good fitting shoe, is probably about 75 to 100 road miles, or about a week's wear in constant marching under ordinary conditions. But where the feet are frequently wet the socks will rub through much sooner.

CHAPTER VIII.

THE CARE OF THE SHOES.

It is highly important, in preventing foot injuries, that a good, well fitting shoe, once secured, shall be kept in good condition. This can be accomplished with a little attention.

The leather of shoes which are put away without use in dry weather tends to become hard and wrinkled. Shoes which are being kept for marching should therefore be worn now and then; and if not sufficiently supple, lightly rubbed over with the neatsfoot oil supplied by the Quartermaster's Department. This oil is the natural oil of the animal and is free from the acids and other substances deleterious to leather found in waxes and greases of other kinds.

In damp, hot weather, as in the tropics, shoes rapidly become covered with mould, which soon destroys the life of the leather and weakens and rots it. Under such conditions, the mould must frequently be thoroughly brushed off and the shoes dried out and the remaining spores or seeds of the mould killed by exposure to the sun. Rubbing with neatsfoot oil also tends to keep down the mould.

Shoes which have been wet must not be put away in that condition, as the leather will shrink out of its original shape into one no longer following the conformation of the foot of the wearer; while hard wrinkles are also formed which are apt to cause blisters and excoriations, especially over the toes. This possible shrinkage has, by test, been found to amount to approximately three-quarters of an inch in the upper of the soldier's shoe. Wet shoes should therefore be carefully dried out; but this drying should not be too rapid or it will harden the leather, and hence care should be used if the shoes are being dried in the sun or before a fire.

When nearly dry, the shoe should be thoroughly brushed or rubbed to remove all dirt and supple the leather. If there is any tendency to stiffness of the leather when completely dry, it should be rubbed again and, if necessary, wiped off with a slightly oiled cloth.

Salt water and alkali water rot the leather and stitching, especially the latter which soon breaks. Shoes soaked in such water should be well washed in fresh water to dissolve out and remove the mineral as soon as possible, and then treated like an ordinary wet shoe.

In the absence of the neatsfoot oil supplied by the Quartermaster's Department, men sometimes rub bacon rind over their shoes to grease them. If this is necessary, the bacon rind must be soaked in several changes of water for several hours to dissolve out the contained salt. But bacon fat used for this purpose soon grows rancid and bad smelling, and attracts flies in warm weather. Unsalted beef tallow from the company kitchen is also good for this purpose; or vaseline, lanolin, or even castor oil, obtained from the Medical Department, may be effectively employed.

In prolonged marching, the inside of shoes is apt to become dirty and sweat soaked. Hence, in addition to the daily use of clean socks, it is well occasionally to wipe out the inside of the shoes with a damp cloth or sponge, and thus remove accumulations of dirt and sweat.

Strong, serviceable and broad shoe lacings must be kept in the shoes at all times. Broken, knotted shoe laces are apt to cause chafing over the instep. In the military shoe, snug lacing is absolutely necessary to hold the shoe in its proper relation to the foot and keep it from slipping around and thus producing blisters, especially over the heel. An extra pair of shoe laces should habitually be carried on the march. In emergency, the lacings of the breeches legs may be used as shoe laces; but as they are round and small, they may cause injury to the parts with which they come into contact.

Many soldiers, if left to themselves, do not lace up their shoes completely, either through carelessness or broken shoe laces. This must be prevented by appropriate orders and inspection at formations. A badly laced shoe on a march will almost certainly cause foot injury.

In repairing military shoes, care must be taken that the man, particularly if of short stature, does not have the heels built up to a height greater than that in the original shoe. Such high heels of course alter the center of gravity of the body and materially diminish facility for marching. A low heel is necessary for proper marching.

Heel nails sometimes work up and protrude inside the shoe. They are easily gotten at in this region, and may be pounded flat with a hammer, gun-butt, bayonet or smooth stone.

In shoes which have been half soled, the new soles are tacked on with nails, the points of which may ultimately work in and project inside of the shoe (See Fig. 54). In the absence of a hammer and iron last with which to flatten them and turn back their points, a small round stone may be held for this purpose over the nail inside the shoe, while the leather of the upper over this stone is smartly struck with a piece of wood or another stone.

A large amount of oil or grease rubbed into the leather tends to keep out moisture and is valuable for use in rainy weather and over wet roads. To apply it, the dry, clean leather is slightly warmed and the oil is well rubbed in with a rag soaked with it until the degree of saturation of the leather required is reached.

But very heavy oiling of shoes fills up all pores of the leather and interferes with evaporation of perspiration, causing the feet in warm weather to be constantly hot and sweaty, and producing much the same results as would follow the use of a rubber boot. This constant moisture softens the skin of the feet, and tends to cause it to break down more readily in the formation of blisters and abrasions. Only just sufficient oil should thus be used on the shoes, during dry weather, to keep the leather supple. Heavy oiling should not be done except when constant exposure of the shoe to wet is anticipated. It is better to let the feet get thoroughly wet now

Fig. 54

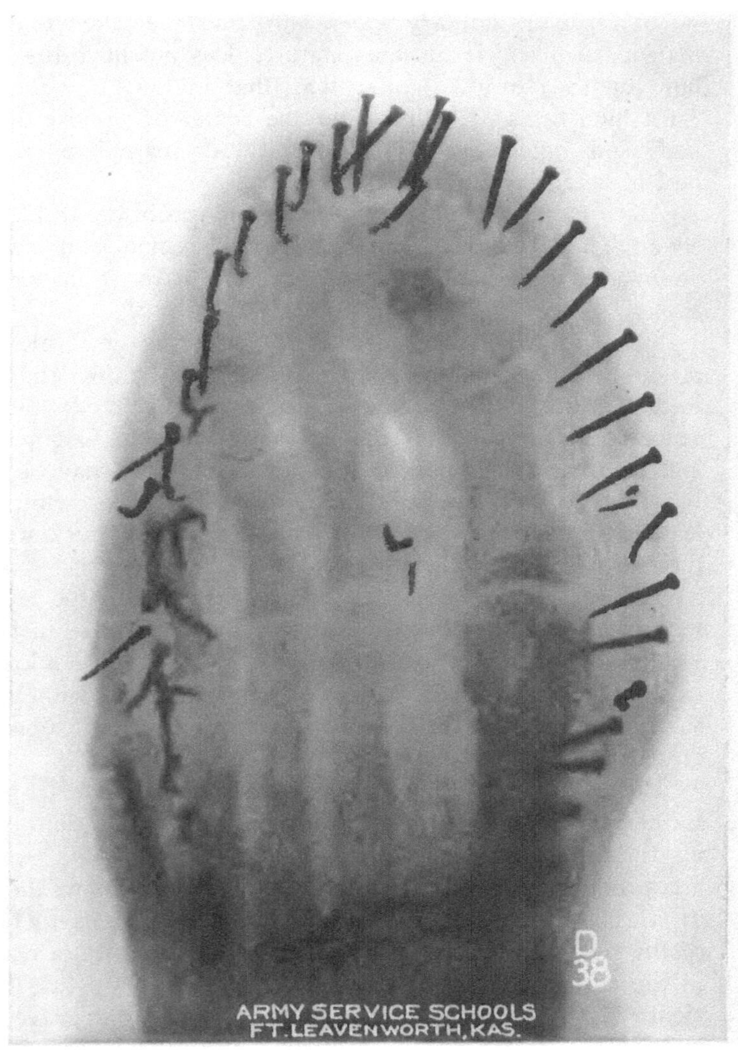

Illustrates the quantity and location of nails used in fastening on a half sole, with their liability to produce foot injury.

and then than to keep them constantly hot and moist by preparation against storms which may be only occasional.

Most prepared waterproof dressings for the shoes contain either wax or paraffine. Both these substances are undesirable, as filling up the pores of the leather and interfering with evaporation of perspiration and hardening the shoe in cold weather. In the French army, a mixture of three parts of mutton tallow to seven parts of neatsfoot oil is used; the proportion of tallow being slightly diminished in cold weather. Tanners generally use a mixture of mutton tallow, cod-liver oil and a little potassium, worked in with a cloth with the aid of gentle heat. Many prepared shoe dressings contain a certain amount of sulphuric acid, which soon induces drying and deterioration of leather and predisposes to cracking, rotting of stitches and entrance of dirt and water.

For working over rough, rocky country, or one with smooth, short grass, hob nails may be driven sparingly into the soles and heels. They give a much better foot-hold on such surfaces and in addition greatly save the sole and heel from wear. But they should not be put in too thickly, as this interferes with the grip of the foot on the ground; nor should they be driven completely through the sole, as they are apt on the one hand to be pressed in and hurt the feet, or on the other to be pulled out and leave holes through which water and sand will enter. The socalled Hungarian hob nail, with a steel head, is best. Smaller hob nails should be put on the heel than on the sole.

The shoes, if damp, must not be used in the field as a head rest at night. This use will press the leather out of shape, and if it dries during the night serious discomfort and possible foot injury may result from wearing such shoes in the morning. The shoes, on being taken off at night, should be worked into their proper shape with the hands and placed on their soles so that the air may have access to their interiors to dry and purify them.

If military conditions are such that the soldier cannot take off his shoes, at least the laces should be loosened so that the feet may be relieved as much as possible from pressure and more air may get to them.

When soldiers are living in tents, the shoes should never be placed in the center, where they are very liable to be trodden upon and pressed out of shape. In barracks, the proper place for shoes in frequent use is under the bunk; for those not in such use, within the man's locker.

In the field, the shoes must be protected from dampness during the night. The shelter tent, poncho or corner of the blanket will protect against rain or dew. But a large amount of dampness also rises from the ground, and to protect against this the shoes should have the poncho or bedding under them, or be raised from the ground by hanging up or by elevation on brush or pieces of wood or stone.

In the field, during freezing weather, the shoes must be carefully dried out by the soldier before going to sleep. Failure to do this will result in a shoe shrunken and hard as horn in the morning, and into which the soldier cannot get his foot until the leather has been thawed out. If the shoes cannot be dried out before bedtime under such conditions, the soldier must keep them on all night or take them to bed with him under his blankets so that they cannot freeze.

If it is desired to dry out shoes rapidly in the field, clean pebbles may be slightly heated in the mess tin over the camp fire, put into the shoe and shaken about in it until the inside moisture has been driven off as vapor. But these pebbles must not be so hot as to injure the leather. Hot, dry cloths stuffed into the shoes, and if necessary re-heated, will also soon absorb any contained moisture.

If wet shoes are packed with dry oats overnight, the oats will absorb the moisture and by their consequent swelling keep the leather of the shoe from shrinking and preserve its proper contour. The oats must be carefully shaken and brushed out of the shoes in the morning, for if any remain they may cause foot injury.

Where a shoe has been wet, and through neglect is subsequently dried out in a way to render it hard and shrunken, the only way in which it can be made immediately available for the march is to sponge off the leather with water until it again becomes soft and yielding to the foot. To march in damp shoes will do no harm; to march in hard, wrinkled and shrunken shoes will almost certainly result in foot injury.

One pair of uppers will usually wear out two sets of soles. When a sole is worn thin, a half sole should be shaped and tacked into position. But no more nails should be used than are necessary to fasten on the half sole firmly, and the nails should be well clinched and pounded smooth inside.

During ordinary campaign, under usual conditions of moisture and roughness of roads as found in this country, a pair of shoes may be expected to last about two months and be sufficient, with light repairs, for a journey of five to six hundred miles over ordinary terrain. But local conditions may very materially modify and reduce this estimate. Rocks and sharp gravel rub away soles rapidly, particularly if wet; while continued wetting for a fortnight or so may cause the stitching to rot and the shoe to fall apart and become unserviceable.

www.ingramcontent.com/pod-product-compliance
Lightning Source LLC
LaVergne TN
LVHW051003080826
845145LV00009B/2431

* 9 7 8 1 4 7 3 3 3 8 1 7 3 *